2-25-9

SEX AND THE HEART

ERECTILE DYSFUNCTION'S LINK TO CARDIOVASCULAR DISEASE

CHRISTOPHER P. STEIDLE, MD
JANET CASPERSON, ANP-C

FOREWORD BY JOHN J. MULCAHY, MD

ADDICUS BOOKS, INC.
OMAHA, NEBRASKA

An Addicus Nonfiction Book

ISBN 978-1-88603996-4

Cover design by Tony Leuenberger and Janice St. Marie
Typography by Linda Dageforde
Illustrations by Coloplast Corp., Advanced Medical Systems, and Jack Kusler.

This book is not intended to serve as a substitute for a physician. Nor is it the authors' intent to give medical advice contrary to that of an attending physician. The authors and publisher disclaim all responsibility for any liability, loss, or risk, personal or otherwise, which may be incurred as a consequence of the use or application of any of the contents of this book.

Library of Congress Cataloging-in-Publication Data
Steidle, Christopher P.
   Sex and the heart :Erectile dysfunction's link to cardiovascular disease / Christopher P. Steidle, Janet Casperson.
      p. cm.
   Includes bibliographical references and index.
   ISBN 978-1-886039-96-4 (alk. paper)
1. Impotence—Popular works. 2. Heart—Diseases—Popular works. I. Casperson, Janet,
   1986- II. Title.

RC889.S686 2008
616.6'92—dc22   2008019343

Addicus Books, Inc.
P.O. Box 45327
Omaha, Nebraska 68145
www.AddicusBooks.com
Printed in the United States of America
10 9 8 7 6 5 4 3 2 1

To our patients, who have shared their stories with us and had the courage to seek treatment for sexual dysfunction, and to the memory of Tony Klee, M.D., anesthesiologist, husband, father, and good friend, whose life ended too soon.

Contents

Acknowledgments

We would like to thank Teresa Brousseau for her help in organizing and putting this book together. We also thank John Mulcahy, M.D., for his steadfast personal and professional support in working to educate health professionals and the public about sexual dysfunction and heart disease.

We also express our gratitude to our patients, who have had the courage to seek treatment for sexual dysfunction despite the fear and the perceived negative connotation associated with it; you have freely shared your stories of health, illness, joy, sadness, successes, failures, sexual intimacy, and romance. We thank you for allowing us to participate in your care and be a part of your lives over the past several years.

Foreword

Erectile dysfunction (ED) is a common problem, affecting up to 30 percent of the male population. The greatest risk factor in the development of ED is aging, and with baby boomers approaching retirement age, the incidence of ED in the population will surely escalate.

The common denominator for both ED and aging is endothelial dysfunction, a condition that occurs when the lining of the blood vessels becomes irregular with the buildup of plaque. This condition is commonly referred to as hardening of the arteries. Some of the first vessels involved in this process are the helicine arteries, which run to the periphery of the erectile bodies in the penis. Blood flowing too slowly from these vessels gives rise to ED, and hence, this symptom may be a harbinger of generalized vascular disease.

The penis is a "barometer" of men's health. When this organ is not functioning properly, it may be a sign that vascular disease in other organs such as the heart and brain may soon follow. In this book, Dr. Christopher Steidle and Janet Casperson, ANP-C, develop this concept in a clear, organized fashion.

They discuss the mechanism of erection and the risk factors contributing to its dysfunction. The relationship between ED and cardiac disease is delineated. When a man presents with ED not associated with surgery or trauma, it would be prudent for him to have a vascular evaluation. This concept is very important since a tremendous number of men will experience ED.

This book is essential reading not only for those with ED, but also for those receiving treatment for vascular diseases such as hypertension, diabetes, and serum lipid abnormalities. The concepts developed in this book are certainly eye-opening.

—John J. Mulcahy, M.D., Ph.D. F.A.C.S.

Introduction

Our purpose in writing this book is to offer a user-friendly resource for couples who are experiencing sexual dysfunction. It was our intent to emphasize and distill the vast amount of scientific research that outlines the profound effects that cardiovascular disease, diabetes, cholesterol abnormalities, and hypertension have on sexual dysfunction, and in particular, erectile dysfunction.

To bring information to the fore, we have relied upon both our clinical experiences in our urology practice and extensive scientific research. Having culled through this research, we can now report on the many risk factors associated with cardiovascular disease and erectile dysfunction. In addition to explaining risk factors and how they develop, we'll discuss appropriate diagnostic evaluations and review treatment options. We hope to give the necessary facts and tools so that you can live a fuller, healthier, and happier life.

PART I

Erectile Dysfunction and Cardiovascular Disease

1

Erectile Dysfunction
and the Heart

The heart is a powerful muscle. Each day, it beats approximately 100,000 times and pumps about two
thousand gallons of blood through miles of vessels
and arteries, delivering oxygen and nutrients to all our vital
organs. Accordingly, our bodies are only as healthy as our
arterial and vascular systems. If these systems are impaired,
the health of all our organs, including the penis, is compromised. In a very real sense, a man's penis is a barometer
of his overall health. There is truth in the adage, "If it's good
for the heart, it's good for the penis."

In fact, medical studies have repeatedly demonstrated
a correlation between cardiovascular disease (CVD) and
sexual dysfunction, specifically erectile dysfunction (ED).

Defining Erectile Dysfunction

Erectile dysfunction is defined as the inability to
achieve or maintain an erection satisfactory for penetration.
If you are unable to maintain an erection until the completion of intercourse, then you probably should be checked
out. You may be asking yourself, "How do I know if I have
erectile dysfunction?" Our response is, "You'll know it when

3

you have it." This is a good way to judge: If you're not having as rigid an erection as you believe you should have, then you have erectile dysfunction.

Overcoming Erectile Dysfunction

Many men ask, "Will I ever be able to have a natural erection again?" The answer to this question is based on the degree of damage that has been done to the tissues of the penis. In men who have relatively new onset of organic erectile dysfunction and who are willing to modify the risk factors, the answer is absolutely yes. However, for men who haven't had a good erection for many years and who have not responded to any of the treatment options, the answer is probably not. However, these men also have viable treatment options, such as penile implants.

Anatomy of the Penis

The penis consists of three columns of tissues surrounded by a thick layer of fascia known as Buck's fascia, covered with subcutaneous tissue and loose skin. The main portion of the penis is made up of a pair of cylinders known as the corpora cavernosa; these cylinders run the length of the penis and have a thick outer membrane called the tunica albuginea. Each of these cylinder bodies communicates with the other through a thin layer of tissues with tiny holes in it.

The erectile tissue itself is basically a bulk of smooth muscle, which is almost pure endothelial tissue. You'll see the term "endothelium" throughout this book. One of the most metabolically active organs in the body, the endothelium makes up the cells that line all the body's blood vessels, including arteries and veins as well as the innermost lining of the penis and other organs.

The urethra, through which we pass urine, is surrounded by a tissue called the corpus spongiosum; it expands at the head, also known as the glans penis. The entire penis has a generous blood supply.

Male Reproductive System

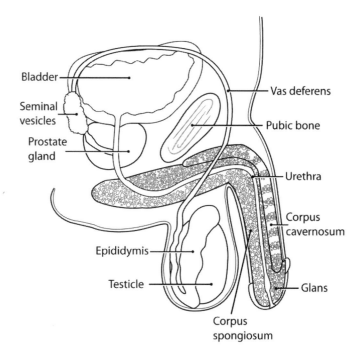

Bladder
Seminal vesicles
Prostate gland
Vas deferens
Pubic bone
Urethra
Corpus cavernosum
Epididymis
Testicle
Glans
Corpus spongiosum

How the Penis Becomes Erect

An erection is a complex event. The process starts with sexually stimulating messages reaching the brain from any of the senses—vision, hearing, smell, taste, or touch. These messages activate nerve centers, which send messages to the erectile tissue in the two cylindrical tissues of the penis. This results in the dilation of the endothelial tissue inside these cylinders, trapping the blood under pressure. Once this occurs, an erection develops.

The real secret to the erection is the relatively newly discovered neurotransmitter called nitric oxide, which is the specific neurotransmitter in the nerve cells that control erections. This discovery is actually what ultimately led to the

Penis Cross Section

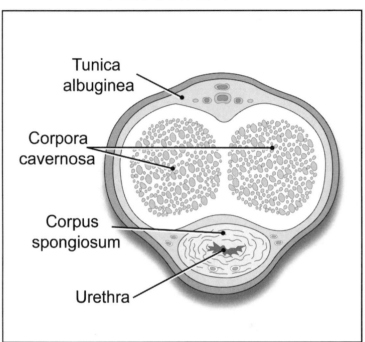

development of the popular erectile dysfunction drugs. Nitric oxide plays a fundamental role in keeping an erection healthy. The reverse is also true, and many men with erectile dysfunction have disorders that decrease the amount of nitric oxide available.

Defining Cardiovascular Disease

Cardiovascular disease is a form of heart disease that results from the narrowing of the coronary arteries that nourish the heart. When they are healthy, these arteries are flexible and have smooth walls; however, over the years, these arteries can become damaged by such things as fats, cholesterol, calcium, cellular debris, and platelets, which are cells that help the blood to clot. When the artery walls are damaged, these substances, called plaque, can stick to them, causing them to gradually clog and become narrowed. The buildup of substances in the arteries is called atherosclerosis, or hardening of the arteries.

Atherosclerosis is the most common form of heart disease in the United States. When the arteries become totally clogged, the result can be a heart attack. Cardiovascular disease is the single largest killer of Americans, claiming a half million lives every year.

Link between Heart Health and Erectile Dysfunction

For the last twenty years, our sexual health clinical practice has focused on the treatment of erectile dysfunction. The connection between cardiovascular disease and erectile dysfunction has changed the way some clinicians view ED. We don't treat only the erectile dysfunction, rather we look for underlying causes of it, such as cardiovascular disease.

It was with the advent of the popular drugs *Viagra, Levitra,* and *Cialis* that our basic understanding of erectile dysfunction began to change dramatically. This realization came about, in part, when Viagra failed in some patients; it led us to focus more on finding other, underlying causes of erectile dysfunction.

In the context of our discussion of sex and heart disease, the abbreviation "ED" can also stand for several key topics, related to erectile dysfunction: early diagnosis, endothelial dysfunction, exercise and diet, effective drugs, and early death.

Early Diagnosis

When a man mentions to his physician that he has erectile dysfunction, he may be saving his own life. Testing for ED may lead to the early diagnosis of cardiovascular disease (CVD). More than 2 million people have coronary disease and have no symptoms; one out of four men with no

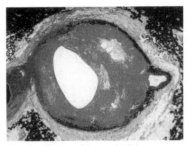
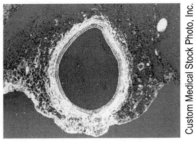

Custom Medical Stock Photo, Inc.

Blocked Artery. Plaque buildup obstructs the flow of blood through this artery. The white area in the center is the only portion of the artery not blocked.

Normal Artery. The open artery, shown above, easily transports oxygenated blood away from the heart and to other parts of the body.

risk factors will die suddenly of a cardiovascular event. It is estimated that more than 50 percent of men with known CVD who underwent vascular surgery had erectile dysfunction. Accordingly, we now view erectile dysfunction as a risk factor and an early indicator of cardiovascular disease.

In a study, published in *Circulation* in 2005, Shlomo Stern, M.D., demonstrated that erectile dysfunction, along with fatigue, shortness of breath, feeling of rapid heartbeat, and genetics, may be potential markers for silent CVD. This is a significant finding.

Endothelial Dysfunction

Endothelial dysfunction is the basis of erectile dysfunction. When the endothelium, tissue that lines the penis, is damaged by such things as diet, tobacco use, and certain lifestyle habits, its performance is affected. Endothelial dysfunction affects the vascular smooth muscle cells, which produce relaxation or contraction, thus affecting the dilation or constriction of blood vessels. When this dysfunction occurs, the arteries, the heart, and other endothelial-lined organs can become hard and stiff. This leads to both coronary artery disease and erectile dysfunction, specifically the inability to maintain an erection adequate for sexual intercourse. The symptom of erectile dysfunction may precede coronary artery disease by as much as four years.

Exercise and Diet

Exercise and diet are one way to insure endothelial health as well as overall health. Exercise and diet are also one of the best treatments for erectile dysfunction, although, unfortunately, it's typically the treatment least used by most men. Still, studies have shown that exercising and losing weight not only can prevent erectile dysfunction but also can actually reverse it.

The Endothelium

The endothelium, the metabolically active tissue that lines the entire circulatory system, is considered the body's largest organ. Weighing nearly five pounds, it is comprised of more than 14,000 square feet of surface area, which would cover the surface area of six and half tennis courts.

Effective Drugs

Not since the approval of birth control pills, which sparked the first sexual revolution of the 1960s, has a single pill—Viagra—made such an impact on society.

With the 1998 release of Viagra, soon followed by Levitra and Cialis, we entered into a second sexual revolution. Never before have we had as many effective drugs available for the treatment of mild to moderate erectile dysfunction. Medically, these drugs are known as PDE-5 inhibitors, which stands for phosphodiesterase type 5 inhibitors. (Throughout this book we will often refer to these three drugs—Viagra, Levitra, Cialis—collectively as PDE-5 inhibitors.)

9

Bob's Story

Our patient Bob is a good example of how treatment for ED has improved over the last two decades. He was in his fifties when he first came to us in 1990 with mild ED. He had been a heavy smoker but was trying to give up the habit. He was overweight and was on medications for high cholesterol; however, he had not altered his eating habits and ate too many fatty foods.

At the time, there were no ED drugs, such as Viagra, available. We taught Bob to give himself penile injections, and he was pleased with the results.

Today, however, we would treat a patient like Bob much differently. Instead of focusing only on helping him achieve an erection, we would have evaluated his risk for cardiovascular disease and related conditions. We would have also checked his blood sugar levels because he was at high risk for Type II Diabetes. In short, Bob was developing a serious condition, which was an underlying factor in his ED.

However, as effective as these drugs are, it is no longer appropriate for us, as clinicians, to prescribe these ED drugs without first questioning a patient about cardiovascular risk factors. When appropriate, we perform a cardiovascular evaluation and, often, other tests to measure for abnormalities in cholesterol levels, blood glucose, and blood pressure; these conditions can affect erectile function on a long-term basis.

Early Death

Unfortunately, early death could result from ignoring endothelial dysfunction and coronary artery disease. American men have nearly a 50 percent chance of dying of cardiovascular disease, and half of these men will die suddenly without any prior warning. Fortunately, we can detect silent heart disease with thorough medical exams; we also now know that men who cannot maintain an erection sufficient for penetration may have significant underlying cardiovascular disease.

2

Overview: Risk Factors for Heart Disease and Erectile Dysfunction

The concept of addressing cardiovascular risk factors in the field of urology and erectile dysfunction is relatively new and extremely important. It's clear now that the risk factors for cardiovascular disease are similar to the risk factors for erectile dysfunction. Any man who is showing signs of erectile dysfunction should be evaluated for underlying cardiovascular disease.

Aging

Aging is the most significant risk factor shared by patients with sexual dysfunction and cardiovascular disease. As men age, the blood flow to the tissues in the penis decreases. This decreased blood flow can lead to a man's inability to achieve and/or maintain an erection.

The concept of aging and risk factors for heart disease is well documented in the Massachusetts Male Aging Study, conducted from 1987 through 1989 among 1,200 randomly selected Boston men, ages forty to seventy. The study examined many facets of the men's health, including their cholesterol levels, blood pressure, lifestyle habits, medications, the presence of heart disease, whether or not they smoked, testosterone levels, and erectile function.

The Massachusetts study found that more than 50 percent of men ages forty to seventy had minimal, moderate, or severe degrees of erectile dysfunction. Age was the factor most strongly associated with erectile dysfunction. The older the man, the more likely he was to have some degree of erectile dysfunction.

The study findings also showed a direct correlation between erectile dysfunction and heart disease, hypertension, diabetes, certain medications, depression, cholesterol levels, smoking, testosterone levels, and personality characteristics.

Cardiovascular and Erectile Dysfunction Risk Factors

Cardiovascular Disease	Erectile Dysfunction
Age	Age
Smoking	Smoking
Obesity	Obesity
Diabetes	Diabetes
High Cholesterol	High Cholesterol
High Blood Pressure (hypertension)	High Blood Pressure (hypertension)
	Testosterone
	Stress
	Depression
	Excessive Alcohol Intake
	Medications (including herbals)
	Prostate Disease
	Relationship Problems
	Neurological Disorders

The Massachusetts study was the first to document the prevalence of erectile dysfunction in America. The study determined that more than 35 million men in America had some level of erectile dysfunction. It was this finding that identified the large market for the PDE-5 inhibitors to treat erectile dysfunction.

The study has been the catalyst for numerous subsequent studies on the aging process in men, and clinicians have gained a great deal of information about this process and how it relates to erectile dysfunction. However, older men can be treated successfully for ED. It's not uncommon in our practice to see many men well into their eighties who have very active sex lives and the desire to keep it that way.

Obesity

Obesity is now the most preventable cause of disease in America. It is a significant risk factor for cardiovascular disease and erectile dysfunction. Obesity is defined as being at a weight greater than 20 percent above the recommended weight for height and age. As a culture, we Americans have progressively gained weight over the last few decades. In 1962, the nation's obesity rate was 13 percent. Now, the Centers for Disease Control reports that 63 percent of Americans are either overweight or obese. Obesity is the cause of nearly 300,000 deaths annually.

Humans weren't always overweight. Many hundreds of years ago, when we were "hunters and gatherers," we didn't eat every day. We lived on very low-calorie diets, and our bodies adapted to long periods of fasting when food was not available. But modern times and technology have given Western nations an abundance of foods available at all times. We eat every day and often excessively. This behavior has contributed to an obesity epidemic. An Italian study documented that even modest weight loss can restore erectile function; we have seen this fact proven in our clinical practice over and over again.

Metabolic Syndrome

Metabolic syndrome, closely related to obesity, is a relatively new condition that we are just beginning to understand. This syndrome is not a single disease, but rather, a cluster of metabolic disorders, which include obesity, insulin resistance, abnormal cholesterol levels, and high blood pressure. According to the National Cholesterol Education Program of the National Heart, Lung, and Blood Institute, you have metabolic syndrome if you have three or more of the criteria listed below.

Criteria for Metabolic Syndrome

- A waistline (measured across the belly) of forty inches or more for men and thirty-five inches or more for women
- A triglyceride level above 150 mg/dL
- High blood pressure (blood pressure of 130/85 mm Hg or higher)
- A fasting blood glucose (sugar) level greater than 100 mg/dL
- A high-density lipoprotein level (HDL) less than 40 mg/dL in men or less than 50 mg/dL in women

---

Measurements are expressed in milligrams per liter of blood.

Metabolic syndrome is made even more complex by the fact that the disorders are interrelated. For example, insulin resistance can cause abnormal blood fats (cholesterol), high blood pressure, and high blood sugar. Similarly, high blood sugar levels can cause abnormal cholesterol levels.

There is recent research that shows when one has metabolic syndrome, belly fat, also called visceral fat, is especially harmful. This fat actually acts almost as a separate organ system and contains cells known as adipocytes that release fatty acids and other hormones into the blood, increasing insulin resistance. When you are insulin resistant, your body does not use insulin effectively so your body pro-

15

duces more. When more insulin is released, appetite is increased, we eat more, and we gain more weight. It becomes a vicious cycle. The fat cells in the abdomen also release toxic chemicals, called cytokines, which disrupt the production of insulin and may promote inflammation of the tissues lining the blood vessels.

Individuals with metabolic syndrome are 3.5 times more likely to die of a heart-related problem and 5 times more likely to develop Type II Diabetes. Men with metabolic syndrome are at much greater risk for erectile dysfunction.

Estimates suggest that approximately 25 percent of the adult population in the United States have metabolic syndrome—that's nearly 55 million people, and many people who are affected don't even know it. Metabolic syndrome is also known by other names such as syndrome X, and insulin resistance syndrome.

Sedentary Lifestyle

Inactivity is a leading contributor to cardiovascular disease, a disease that claims more lives than any other in the United States. Moderate physical activity can significantly lower one's risk for heart disease, Type II Diabetes, and certain cancers, including colon cancer. Exercise also reduces blood pressure and cholesterol levels and helps with weight management. All of these factors affect erectile dysfunction.

Unfortunately, only about 30 percent of Americans exercise regularly. (Adequate exercise is considered to be at least thirty minutes of physical activity three to five times a week.)

Smoking

Tobacco use is one of our health's greatest enemies. Smoking is responsible for more than 400,000 deaths per year, making tobacco use the leading cause of preventable disability and death. Although the numbers of smokers are declining, millions of Americans continue to smoke. The detrimental effects of tobacco use include: cancer, hypertension, lung disease, asthma, allergies, heart disease, strokes, increased heart rate, shortness of breath, bladder and kidney disorders, digestive diseases, poor physical fitness, sexual dysfunction, and erectile dysfunction.

We have often speculated what might happen if manufacturers put the following message on the side of a cigarette package: "Warning: Smoking Will Cause Loss of Erections." We believe few men would continue smoking if they saw this warning.

Random studies that examine the effects of smoking on erections and sexual dysfunction have not been well detailed in the medical literature. But through our years of clinical practice, we have learned that tobacco affects both the quality and rigidity of erections. We have seen severe end-stage erectile dysfunction in men with a long history of heavy smoking. It is worth repeating that smoking is one of the biggest risk factors for both cardiovascular disease and erectile dysfunction.

Diabetes

Diabetes is a disease in which the body does not produce or properly use insulin. Insulin is a hormone that is needed to convert sugar, starches, and other food into energy needed for daily life. Without proper regulation, blood sugars rise. Diabetes, if left uncontrolled, leads to very serious health problems—65 percent of people with diabetes die from heart attacks or strokes, according to the American Diabetes Association.

It is estimated that nearly 21 million Americans have diabetes; approximately 6 million of them have never been diagnosed. Diabetes is categorized into two types: Type I Diabetes, also referred to as juvenile diabetes, and Type II Diabetes.

Dyslipidemia (Abnormal Cholesterol Levels)

In the simplest terms, dyslipidemia refers to having abnormally high levels of fats, or cholesterol, in the blood. If left untreated, a buildup of these fats can cause a form of heart disease known as atherosclerosis, in which the artery walls become blocked with fatty deposits. The condition can lead to a stroke if blood vessels leading to the brain or neck become clogged. Dyslipidemia can also cause blockages in vessels going to the legs; this can result in the need for amputations. It is understandable that such interruptions in blood flow can also affect a man's ability to get an erection.

According to the American Heart Association, nearly 107 million Americans have elevated cholesterol levels. Of this number, 37 million have dangerously high levels, putting them at risk for heart attack and strokes, which can be fatal.

Hypertension

Hypertension is the medical term for high blood pressure. An estimated 72 million people, nearly one-third of Americans, have high blood pressure. Unfortunately, as many as 75 percent of these individuals are not aware they have it, and of those who know they have it, 64 percent do not keep the disease under control.

High blood pressure can lead to both heart attacks and stroke. Hypertension causes erectile dysfunction in at-risk individuals, but oftentimes, the treatment for hypertension negatively affects erections, arousal, and the ability to achieve orgasm as well.

Causes of Erectile Dysfunction Not Related to the Heart

Low Testosterone Levels

Having low testosterone levels is known as hypogonadism. It is a common condition associated with both diabetes and a high body mass index (BMI) or obesity. Testosterone levels will be discussed in detail in chapter 6.

Neurogenic Causes

Neurogenic causes of erectile dysfunction are those that are caused by nerve damage. These less-common risk factors for ED damage the nerves that supply the penis; this damage can cause changes such as in sensation and/or numbness in the glans, or head of the penis. Neurological risk factors include multiple sclerosis, spinal cord injury, non-nerve-sparing surgery within the pelvis, pelvic injury, stroke, epilepsy, Parkinson's disease, brain tumors, Alzheimer's disease, and head trauma.

Another cause of neurogenic damage is alcoholic neuropathy, which can result from the consumption of excessive amounts of alcohol over an extended period of time. The condition may cause numbness and loss of sensation in the lower extremities, including the penis. Also, examination of patients with alcoholic neuropathy typically reveals very small testicles.

One of the newly identified risk factors for neurologic damage is bicycle seat configuration. It has been documented that certain types of bicycle seats used by men who do distance riding can affect erectile dysfunction by damaging the nerves and arteries to the penis, causing a low blood flow.

Prostate Disease

Prostate disease can affect erectile dysfunction. Men who have undergone a radical prostatectomy (removal of the prostate gland) may experience ED. The risk of impotence for men who have had a prostatectomy is about 30 percent for men in their forties and rises with age to about 80 percent for men in their seventies.

Endocrinologic Causes

Endocrinologic causes of erectile dysfunction include hypogonadism (low testosterone), pituitary tumors, and rare congenital conditions such as Klinefelter syndrome, a chromosomal abnormality marked by the presence of an extra sex hormone. Males with Klinefelter syndrome have an XXY chromosome instead of the usual XY male chromosome.

Peyronie's Disease

Peyronie's disease refers to scar tissue or plaque in the erectile tissue in the penis, sometimes causing painful and curved erections. The condition may develop slowly over time, or the symptoms may develop rapidly. Symptoms may include hardened scar tissue in the penis, pain during erections, curvature or bend in the penis when erect, narrowing of the diameter of the penis when erect, and erectile dysfunction. The scarring may occur on the top or bottom of the penis; it can also occur on both sides of the penis.

Kidney Deficiency

Chronic kidney deficiency places a man at higher risk for erectile dysfunction due to blood-flow conditions and low testosterone. These may be a consequence of the conditions that are associated with renal failure, including anemia, depression, protein deficiency, high blood pressure, and the use of antihypertensive medications.

Measuring the patient's creatinine and kidney function is important when treating a man with erectile dysfunction who is on dialysis or who has chronic renal deficiencies. The measurements are used to determine the correct dosage of either PDE-5 inhibitors or injection therapy and prevent an overdose, which can lead to priapism or damaging metabolic effects.

Psychological Factors in ED

The fact that stress is a risk factor for erectile dysfunction is no surprise, given life in modern America. A million years ago, human stress was related to protecting yourself from wild animals. The stress response is known as a sympathetic discharge—the sympathetic nervous system releases the hormone called cortisol. This is the "fight-or-flight" hormone, which allows humans to face a situation or run away from it. When cortisol is released, it causes an increase in blood pressure, increased blood flow to organs that are needed for rapid activity, increased mental activity, increased blood glucose, and an increased metabolic rate. It decreases blood flow to organs not needed for rapid activity.

The sex organs are not vital for rapid activity and therefore receive less of the blood flow. One way to understand this response is to imagine someone walking in on you when you're in the midst of sexual activity. What's the first thing that happens? Usually, a loss of an erection. This is a sympathetic event. You are startled, you have a "fight-or-flight" response, and your body releases cortisol. Blood flow is diverted from the sex organs.

Unfortunately, today the stress in our life may be in the boardroom, in the office, or on the highway. The stress isn't met with aggressive physical activity output, but the stress is real and constant nonetheless. Cortisol levels become too high, and glands become exhausted. The way you handle stress can dramatically affect erectile dysfunction.

Relationship problems can be complex. We all understand that "it takes two to tango," and a poor or strained relationship can affect a man's ability to become erect. It's important to work on your relationship at the same time you work on modifying risk factors.

In Summary

In conclusion, the relationship between cardiovascular disease and erectile dysfunction is well documented by research. CVD and ED share many of the same risk factors, some of which can be modified. Remember, to paraphrase the old adage mentioned earlier, "If it is going to make your heart healthier, it is going to make your sex life healthier."

PART II

Conditions Related to Heart Disease and Erectile Dysfunction

3

Diabetes

As mentioned earlier, diabetes is a risk factor for both cardiovascular disease and erectile dysfunction. In this chapter, we'll take a closer look at diabetes.

One important study examined the relationship between diabetes, heart disease, and ED. The study involved two groups of men. The first group consisted of men with diabetes who *were* able to maintain their erections. These men had no greater risk of having a silent heart attack than men in the general population.

The second group was made up of men with diabetes who *could not* maintain erections. These men were eight times more likely to have a silent cardiovascular event than the men in the first group. This is a profound finding. The loss of maintenance of the erection in a man with diabetes is a harbinger of silent cardiovascular disease and should not be ignored.

Type I Diabetes

Type I Diabetes accounts for about 5 to 10 percent of diagnosed diabetes in the United States; it develops most often in children and young adults but can appear at any age. Type I Diabetes is an autoimmune disease, which results when the body's system for fighting infection, the immune system, turns against the body and destroys the beta cells in the pancreas. These cells produce insulin and regulate our blood-sugar balance. When they are destroyed, the body's ability to maintain a balance of insulin and blood sugars is altered. With the death of beta cells in the pancreas, the body has no insulin and is therefore unable to process foods properly and the blood sugars increase. It's not completely understood why the body's immune system attacks the beta cells, but several factors are probably involved, including autoimmune response, genetics, environmental conditions, and possibly viruses.

Men with Type I Diabetes have an earlier onset and a more-severe degree of sexual dysfunction, and they are generally less responsive to conservative medical treatment. Additionally, most of the men who develop Type I Diabetes usually do so in their early teens, often before they are sexually active. So, by the time they begin to have sexual activity, the disease is typically more advanced.

Type I diabetics need daily injections of insulin, which controls the disease. Before the discovery of insulin, people often died from diabetes. Unfortunately, controlling Type II Diabetes is not that simple, and people diagnosed with it must make a concerted effort to make changes in their lives in order to bring the disease under control.

Fasting Blood-Sugar-Level Classifications

Normal	Less than 100 mg/dL
Diabetes	Greater than 125 mg/dL

Measurements are expressed in milligrams per liter of blood.

Type II Diabetes

Much more common than Type I Diabetes, Type II Diabetes accounts for about 90 to 95 percent of diabetes cases in the United States. This form of diabetes is most often associated with older age, obesity, family history of diabetes, previous history of physical inactivity, and African American ethnicity.

With Type II Diabetes, the pancreas is usually producing enough insulin, but for unknown reasons, the body cannot use the insulin effectively, a condition called insulin resistance. Essentially, the body is resisting the use of its own insulin. After several years, this causes a decrease in the production of insulin. As a result, glucose, the body's main source of fuel, builds up in the blood and cannot be used efficiently. We know obesity is a factor in insulin resistance; most people develop the condition when they become 30 percent or more overweight. About 80 percent of people with Type II Diabetes are overweight.

How Diabetes Causes Erectile Dysfunction

Erectile dysfunction is a common complication of diabetes. In fact, sexual dysfunction may be the symptom that causes a man to seek health care, which, in turn, leads to a diagnosis of the diabetes. The prevalence of erectile dysfunction in men with diabetes is 5 to 75 percent; at age sixty, that number is reported to be anywhere from 55 to 95 percent.

Decreased desire, and decreased orgasmic function, as well as the inability to achieve and maintain an erection, may mark the onset of sexual dysfunction in men. In men with diabetes, this occurs within five to ten years from the onset of the disease and increases with age if the disease is not brought under control.

Often, we see a more-significant degree of erectile dysfunction in men with diabetes because many men with Type II Diabetes had the disease for at least a decade and did not know it. Why is sexual dysfunction more severe and more challenging to treat in our patients who have diabetes? Recently, more resources have been given to study this phenomenon and the results are both astounding and complex. At the root of the problem is endothelial dysfunction.

Unfortunately, in patients with diabetes, endothelial dysfunction is manifested in many different ways that can cause not only erectile dysfunction but also other diseases related to diabetes. These other diseases may include: heart disease, obesity, hormonal imbalances, stress, hypertension, dyslipidemia, gonadal dysfunction, depression, and neuropathy.

Age, a sedentary lifestyle, and tobacco use further increase the risk of sexual dysfunction. Any of these factors can be the cause of erectile dysfunction by themselves, but when they occur with compromised endothelial integrity, the negative effects are strengthened. If the effects are profound, the symptoms may be irreversible.

Diabetic Neuropathy

All men who develop diabetic neuropathy, a common complication of diabetes in which nerves are damaged as a result of high blood-sugar levels, will have some form and degree of erectile dysfunction. The earliest signs and symptom of diabetic neuropathy is the loss of vibratory sensation in the feet. The penis and the feet share a similar neurologic pathway. Accordingly, the penis can lose sensation also.

Low Testosterone and Diabetes

For several reasons, hypogonadism, having low testosterone levels, is an extremely common condition in men with diabetes. Probably the biggest reason is the increased weight and increased levels of a protein called sex hormone binding globulin (SHBG) in the bloodstream. The SHBG binds up the body's available testosterone, so the available levels are lower; this leads to a cycle in which the low testosterone levels thwart a man's ability to lose weight, so weight often increases, further causing the SHBG to bind up yet more of the testosterone. As the cycle continues, the man continues to gain weight.

Several recent studies have demonstrated that erectile dysfunction is much more successfully treated when testosterone is at optimal levels. This is particularly true for a patient with diabetes. It is not uncommon for us to see men who have a poor response to PDE-5 inhibitors respond dramatically positively when they are treated with testosterone. There is a very specific reason for this: the enzyme needed for PDE-5 inhibitors to work is called nitric oxide. This substance depends on the presence of testosterone for production. So, when there is no nitric oxide, ED drugs do not work.

Hemoglobin A1c Test

Blood testing is a very important component of the workup for diabetes and erectile dysfunction. An important blood test, the hemoglobin A1c test, calculates blood sugar levels over the last three to four months. Hemoglobin A1c is a blood protein in red blood cells that bonds with blood sugar. Since red blood cells can live from 90 to 120 days, the hemoglobin A1c stays in the blood for that length of time.

Accordingly, it is effective in measuring blood sugar over a period of time. Most clinicians run this test routinely, sometimes as often as every three months, for people with diabetes or metabolic syndrome. A normal A1c level is less than 6 percent hemoglobin A1c. Some doctors prefer an even lower 5.5 percent.

Treating ED in Men with Diabetes

In subsequent chapters, we'll describe standard treatments for ED in detail. However, we'd like to make a few points about treatment for sexual dysfunction in men with diabetes. The treatment for diabetes is dependent on the severity of the diabetes and how far a man is willing to go to restore his ability to be sexually active. Diabetes has some variables that require different approaches with several of the standard treatments.

For example, primary treatment is aimed at preventing and controlling the diabetes with both lifestyle modifications and medications for erectile function. This treatment centers around a multidisciplinary approach to maintaining tight control of blood sugar levels and other factors such as high cholesterol, hypertension, and hypogonadism (low testosterone). Controlling blood sugar levels means that patients must carefully manage their diabetes so their blood sugars are maintained in a relatively tight range.

But diabetes is not just about blood sugar. Diabetes also contributes to cardiovascular disease, affects cholesterol levels, and can contribute to obesity. It's also well documented that diabetes is a leading cause of endothelial dysfunction, which causes inflammation of the heart.

In many diabetics, the disease has progressed to the point that the tissues are unresponsive to lower doses of ED medications alone. In these cases, we often use a combination of therapies to treat erectile dysfunction. In our clinical practice, we frequently use higher doses of testosterone and PDE-5 inhibitors or penile injections in men with diabetes in order to achieve patient and partner satisfaction.

Penile implant surgery is frequently used with great success in men with diabetes and severe erectile dysfunction. The biggest risk of this surgery is infection. However, with tight glycemic control, which is defined as an A1c of less than 7, the risk for infection decreases dramatically.

We now know that abnormal cholesterol levels and high blood pressure are directly associated with diabetes; however, these can be managed. The most important key here is education for the patient.

Medications for Diabetes

The most popular drug prescribed for diabetes is metformin; it works by reducing the liver's natural production of sugar and by improving insulin sensitivity. This drug is marketed as *Glucophage, Glucophage XR,* and generic versions. Other commonly prescribed drugs include: rosiglitazone *(Avandia)*, pioglitazone *(Actos)*, metformin and rosiglitazone *(Avandamet)*, exenatide *(Byetta)*, pramlintide *(Symlin)*, and sitagliptin *(Januvia)*.

In Summary

Successful management of cardiovascular disease and erectile or sexual dysfunction for the patient with diabetes is based on the control of the diabetes disease process. Maintaining tight glycemic control is the primary key to successful management of diabetes. Never before has there been more information, medications, and treatments available for treating this disease. A decade ago, patients did not regularly have access to glucose meters. Now, patients commonly are able to check their sugar three or four times a day, carefully monitor their intake of carbohydrates, and measure their three-month average of blood sugar.

It's important to remember that primary prevention, if aggressively maintained, will stop the progression of erectile dysfunction. If men do not modify the primary cause of erectile dysfunction, such as diabetes or uncontrolled hypertension, the medications for erectile dysfunction will eventually cease to work. Finally, remember that the loss of an erection in a man with diabetes is a harbinger of silent cardiovascular disease and should not be ignored.

4

Dyslipidemia

Dyslipidemia is a condition marked by abnormally high concentrations of lipids, or cholesterol, in the blood. What is cholesterol? It is a waxy substance found in all our cells; it is necessary for life and helps us digest fats, it strengthens cell membranes, and it makes some hormones and vitamins. Cholesterol moves through the bloodstream; however, it cannot dissolve in the blood. So, when too much of it builds up in our arteries, it forms a substance called plaque, which clogs arteries and restricts blood flow. High cholesterol is a significant risk factor in developing cardiovascular disease.

The particles that carry cholesterol through the bloodstream are called lipoproteins. You are probably most familiar with lipoproteins being referred to as: low- density lipoprotein (LDL), high-density lipoprotein (HDL), triglycerides, and very-low-density lipoprotein (VLDL).

How High Cholesterol Causes ED

It has been well documented that high lipids, or high total cholesterol, are commonly associated with erectile dysfunction. In many men with ED, high cholesterol levels, known as hypercholesterolemia, is the only risk factor seen. If high cholesterol creates a buildup of plaque in the arteries, the flow of blood can be impaired to any number of organs, including the sex organs. The lack of inflow of blood into the penis results in diminished erections.

The Massachusetts Male Aging Study found that elevation of HDL is associated with longevity and preservation of erectile dysfunction no matter the age, whereas elevation of LDL is associated with early cardiovascular disease and early erectile dysfunction.

Factors Affecting Cholesterol Levels

We get cholesterol in two ways—from the liver naturally and from the foods we eat. Other factors also affect cholesterol levels, including diet, weight, exercise, heredity, age, and gender. Of these, we can control diet, weight, and exercise. An atherogenic diet, also called the Standard American Diet, which contains too much dietary cholesterol and saturated fat and too little polyunsaturated fat, is known to promote plaque formation and early atherosclerosis.

Our bodies need healthful fats such as olive oil and canola oil to manufacture the necessary hormones for the correct functioning of the body. But eating saturated fat such as that found in animal products, especially fatty red meats; eggs; palm oil; and coconut oil also contributes to the elevation of LDL or low-density lipoproteins, the "lethal" cholesterol. Such an unhealthful diet is strongly associated with erectile dysfunction.

Testing Cholesterol Levels

The published guidelines for lipid disorder management are well known by primary care physicians and specialists. The blood test for a total cholesterol level measures blood cholesterol in all lipoproteins combined. Men with a total cholesterol greater than 240 mg/dL have a 2.7-fold increased risk for having moderate to severe erectile dysfunction. This makes an elevated serum cholesterol one of the most important risk factors for the subsequent development of erectile dysfunction.

Total Cholesterol (TC) Levels

Desirable	less than 200 mg/dL
Borderline high	200–239 mg/dL
High	240 mg/dL and above

Measurements are expressed in milligrams per liter of blood.

LDL Cholesterol

Low-density lipoprotein (LDL) cholesterol is sometimes called "bad" cholesterol. An easy way to remember that LDL is the bad cholesterol is to think of the "L" as standing for the "lethal" cholesterol. The higher the LDL level in your blood, the greater the chance that your arteries will become clogged and you will develop heart disease. The goal is to have low levels of LDL.

LDL Cholesterol Levels

Ideal	less than 70 mg/dL
Normal	70–100 mg/dL
Borderline High	100–130 mg/dL
High	130–160 mg/dL
Very High	greater than 160 mg/dL

Measurements are expressed in milligrams per liter of blood.

HDL Cholesterol

High-density lipoprotein (HDL) cholesterol is sometimes called "good" cholesterol or "healthful" cholesterol. It carries cholesterol from other parts of your body back to your liver, where it is removed from your body. The higher your HDL cholesterol level, the lower your chance of getting heart disease.

HDL Cholesterol Levels

High	60 mg/dL (desired level)
Low	less than 40 mg/dL

Measurements are expressed in milligrams per liter of blood.

Triglycerides

Most of the fat in the body is made up of triglycerides, which are stored in the body's fat tissues. When the body needs energy, these fat tissues break down the triglycerides and release them into the bloodstream as fatty acids.

Triglycerides are the most common form of fat in your diet. The majority of the fats you eat, including vegetable oil and animal products, contain triglycerides. Also, carbohydrates are converted to triglycerides by the body. When you eat more than you need, the body converts the excess calories to triglycerides, which are then stored as fat.

Triglyceride Levels

Normal	less than 150 mg/dL
High	150–199 mg/dL
Very High	200–499 mg/dL
Extremely High	greater than 500 mg/dL

Measurements are expressed in milligrams per liter of blood.

VLDL

The very-low-density lipoprotein (VLDL) cholesterol contains about 15 percent of the blood's cholesterol and most of the triglycerides. A significant amount of VLDL is converted to LDL cholesterol. Consequently, some types of

35

VLDL cholesterol may contribute to plaque building. Normal VLDL levels are between 5 and 40 mg/dL.

Medications Used to Treat Cholesterol Disorders

The guidelines for treating abnormal cholesterol levels emphasize therapeutic lifestyle modifications focusing on exercise, diet, weight loss, and, of course, smoking cessation as the cornerstones of care. We'll cover these modifications in chapter 11. If these aggressive lifestyle modifications are not successful, then drug management should be introduced. The primary goal is to decrease LDL, the "bad" cholesterol, with the target being an LDL level of less than 100 mg/dL.

There are many common and effective medications for treating lipid disorders. They need to be used in combination with a balanced, nutritional diet and an exercise plan.

Statins

Widely used and effective, a class of drugs called statins are the gold standard for treatment of lipid disorders. Among the best-selling drugs in U.S. history, statins help the body get rid of cholesterol. How do statins work? They inhibit an enzyme in the liver needed by the body to manufacture cholesterol. Statins have some side effects but are generally very safe and very well tolerated.

What is important about statins is that several studies have shown that treatment with statins, particularly atorvastatin (*Lipitor*), can improve sexual function and the response to the PDE-5 inhibitors in men who do not respond to the PDE-5 inhibitors alone. A pilot study supported the concept that statins can help improve endothelial function, the primary defect seen with erectile dysfunction.

Commonly prescribed statins include: atorvastatin (*Lipitor*), fluvastatin (*Lescol*), lovastatin (*Mevacor*), pravastatin (*Pravachol*), rosuvastatin (*Crestor*), and simvastatin (*Zocor*).

Ezetimibe (Zetia)

One new medication used in the treatment of high cholesterol is a cholesterol absorption inhibitor that interferes with the absorption of cholesterol in the digestive tract. This drug is marketed as *Zetia*.

Fibrates

Often used in combination with statins, fibrates affect fatty acid metabolism and lower triglycerides, often by as much as 20 to 50 percent. They also can boost the good cholesterol, HDL, by up to 15 percent. They may have a mild effect on LDL.

Commonly prescribed fibrates include: fenofibrate (*TriCor, Triglide*) and gemfibrozil (*Lopid*).

Nicotinic Acid

Niacin, or nicotinic acid, is one of the oldest drugs used for lowering cholesterol levels. It can help lower LDL and triglycerides while boosting HDL levels. Niacin is relatively well tolerated by most people but may cause some flushing, which is a hot, tingling sensation in the skin, and should be used with caution in patients with diabetes.

Commonly prescribed drugs in this class are: *Niacor* and *Niaspan*. A related drug, *Advicor*, is a combination of niacin and lovastatin.

Bile Acid Sequestrants

Bile acid sequestrants, a class of drugs also known as resins, are an older type of lipid-lowering medication; they work by binding fats in the diet and preventing their absorption, decreasing cholesterol.

Commonly prescribed drugs include: cholestyramine (*Questran*), colestipol (*Colestid*), and colesevelam (*WelChol*).

Omega-3 Fatty Acids

Perhaps one of the best treatments to lower bad cholesterol is also one of the oldest and most natural treatments.

Omega-3 fatty acids, a supplement you can buy over the counter, are typically derived from cold-water fish and other sources. They are becoming more and more popular in combating high cholesterol levels. They have a multitude of positive effects in the human body and are currently recommended for people with high triglyceride levels.

In Summary

It is extremely important to know your lipid profile. Discuss it with your clinician, and manage it with either a therapeutic lifestyle modification or medication or a combination of both. Your lipid metabolism is important to your ability to achieve and maintain an erection. Erectile dysfunction can be one of the earliest symptoms of a lipid disorder and can help facilitate the diagnosis.

Yes, drugs can help, but remember that the drugs currently available for the treatment of erectile dysfunction merely treat the symptom and do nothing to change the underlying causes. We cannot stop the progression of erectile dysfunction without therapeutic lifestyle changes.

5

Hypertension

Hypertension, or high blood pressure, is one of the world's most common health conditions. You may have heard high blood pressure referred to as the "silent killer." That's because it has virtually no symptoms, and many people are not aware that they have it. They may only become aware of it if they develop symptoms such as headaches, dizziness, sleeplessness, or ringing in the ears. More seriously, anyone with high blood pressure is at increased risk for heart attack, sudden death, or stroke.

Blood pressure refers to the force applied to the artery walls as the heart pumps the blood. Moving the blood takes a certain amount of pressure, and as more pressure is needed to pump and circulate blood through our organs, there is potential for this force to also damage organs in our bodies. Unfortunately, hypertension often accompanies metabolic syndrome, diabetes, and other health risk factors. It is the combination of these risk factors together with hypertension that make it a very lethal force.

Measuring Blood Pressure

There are two forms of measurement of blood pressure. Systolic blood pressure is the pressure when the heart beats. The pressure when the heart is resting is known as the diastolic pressure. When your health care professional takes your blood pressure, he/she will list the systolic pressure, which is higher, over the diastolic pressure, which is lower. A normal blood pressure is 120/80 or lower.

Classification of Blood Pressure Levels

	Upper Number	Lower Number
Normal	Systolic below 120	Diastolic below 80
Prehypertension	Systolic 120–139	Diastolic 80-89
Stage 1 hypertension	Systolic 140–159	Diastolic 90-99
Stage 2 hypertension	Systolic 160 and higher	Diastolic 100 and higher

How Hypertension Causes ED

Hypertension is the second-most-prevalent concurrent disease in men with erectile dysfunction. When we look at how hypertension causes ED, we again are looking at the function of the endothelium. You'll recall that the endothelium is the layer of cells that lines the interior surface of the body's blood vessels. In the penis, these cells dilate in response to certain signals generated by both hormones and nerve cells to cause an erection. The endothelial cells then relax and allow a seal to be made to prevent blood from leaking out of the penis. Diseases that affect the endothelium, such as hypertension, can prevent this endothelial relaxation which prevents the blood from staying in the penis. We call this condition a venous leak.

How Hypertension Drugs May Cause ED

Unfortunately, the medications that prevent hypertension can also contribute to erectile dysfunction. Why do these drugs cause ED? When beta-blockers lower blood pressure, they're also lowering the pressure of blood flowing into the penis. Beta-blockers may also impair the response to nerve impulses that cause a man to get an erection. These drugs also make it more difficult for the arteries in the penis to widen and take in blood. Also, beta-blockers can bring on a sedated, tired feeling, which may affect a man's becoming aroused.

Unfortunately, when men experience sexual dysfunction as a side effect of antihypertensive medications, they sometimes stop the medication. It's been estimated that as many as 70 percent of hypertensive men who have had significant side effects, particularly side effects related to sexual dysfunction, are noncompliant with their medication. It's important to remember that you should *never* stop taking hypertension drugs without first consulting your physician.

Medications for High Blood Pressure

Drugs known as diuretics are among the medications that are most likely to impair a man's ability to get an erection. As mentioned, beta-blockers can also dramatically affect erections.

Thiazide Diuretics

The thiazide diuretics are the mainstays of high blood pressure drugs. These medications are used alone or, more commonly, as a combination pill. If these drugs cause ED when a man first starts taking them, it's reasonable for the doctor to change the medications. For example, if a man says "I had great erections, but when I started a thiazide diuretic, my erections became bad," the physician will likely change the medication. A man who says "I've been on a thiazide diuretic for twenty years and I've slowly lost my erections," requires a different medication to treat the erectile dysfunction and not just a different diuretic. The specific discussion and decision regarding changing medications should be undertaken between a patient and his health professional who prescribed the antihypertensive medications.

Commonly prescribed diuretics include: hydrochlorthiazide (*HCTZ, Hydodiuril*), chlorthalidone (*Hygroton*), indapamide (*Lozol*), furosemide (*Lasix*), torsemide (*Demedex*), bumetanide (*Bumex*), and metolazone (*Zaroxolyn*).

Beta-Blockers

Beta-blockers are another class of medications that are commonly used alone or in combination with other therapies for men with hypertension. Beta-blockers reduce blood pressure by decreasing heart rate, reducing the strength of the heart's contractions, and relaxing blood vessel walls.

Unfortunately, beta-blockers have a significant association with erectile dysfunction. For this reason, if men complain that their erections were adequate but decreased dramatically when they started a beta-blocker, it is time for a discussion with the health professional who prescribed the medication and perhaps a change of beta-blockers.

Commonly prescribed beta-blockers include: metoprolol (*Lopressor, Toprol XL*), atenolol (*Tenormin*), propranolol (*Inderal*), sotalol (*Betapace*), and timolol (*Blocadren*).

Alpha-Blockers

The alpha-blockers are used for hypertension and more commonly have been used to treat men for the symptoms related to an enlarged prostate. These drugs have not been shown to affect the erection in an adverse way. However, they have been shown to cause retrograde ejaculation, in which semen is not expelled but rather goes into the bladder. Retrograde ejaculation is the reason some men do not like to take alpha-blockers. They are usually not primary therapy for a man with a new diagnosis of hypertension but are more commonly used in combination therapy. A newer class of alpha-blockers formulated specifically for prostate disease does not tend to have as many cardiovascular side effects.

Commonly prescribed alpha-blockers include: doxazosin mesylate *(Cardura)*, prazosin hydrochloride *(Minipress)*, and terazosin hydrochloride *(Hytrin)*. Note: if you are taking an alpha-blocker, *do not mix it* with an ED drug (Viagra, Levitra, or Cialis). *Talk to your doctor first.* We tell our patients to take these medications at least four hours apart.

Calcium Channel Blockers

Another class of medications used in blood pressure management is the calcium channel blocker. These are very common medications which have not been shown to have a dramatic effect on erectile function. They are commonly used alone and are also included in "step therapy," which is used in patients who have difficult-to-treat high blood pressure requiring multiple medications.

Commonly prescribed calcium channel blockers include: diltiazem hydrochloride *(Cardizem, Dilacor, Cartia XT)*, amlodipine besylate *(Norvasc)*, felodipine *(Plendil)*, nimodipine *(Nimotop)*, nifedipine *(Adalat, Procardia)*, nicardipine *(Cardene)*, and verapamil *(Calan, Isoptin, Verelan, Covera)*.

Angiotensin Receptor Blockers (ARBs)

Perhaps the best medication available to treat high blood pressure in men with erectile dysfunction is the angiotensin receptor blockers or ARBs. This class of compounds includes drugs such as valsartan. This medication is one of the few that do not adversely affect erections. Angiotensin receptor blockers are probably the number one choice for use in men who have erection problems related to hypertensive therapy.

Commonly prescribed ARBs include: candesartan cilexitil *(Atacand)*, irbesartan *(Avapro)*, losartan *(Cozaar, Hyzaar)*, olmesartan *(Benicar)*, telmisartan *(Micardis)*, and valsartan *(Diovan)*.

Angiotensin-Converting Enzyme (ACE) Inhibitors

Another class of antihypertensive medication that is particularly useful in men with erectile dysfunction is the angiotensin-converting enzyme (ACE) inhibitor. These drugs block the formation of angiotensin, which causes blood vessels to constrict. These drugs may be used alone or in combination with other drugs.

Commonly prescribed ACEs include: benazepril *(Lotensin)*, captopril *(Capoten)*, fosinopril sodium *(Monopril)*, enalapril *(Vasotec)*, lisinopril *(Prinivil, Zestril)*, ramipril *(Altace)*, quinapril *(Accupril)*, and trandolapril *(Mavik)*, and perindopril erbumine *(Aceon)*.

Prehypertension

The National Heart, Lung, and Blood Institute guidelines for high blood pressure were modified in 2003. Blood pressures previously considered to be within the "normal" range are now considered to be within the "prehypertensive" category.

The guidelines do not recommend drug therapy for those with prehypertension unless it is required for another condition, such as diabetes or chronic kidney disease. But people who are prehypertensive and people with normal blood pressures are encouraged to make therapeutic lifestyle changes including losing excess weight, becoming physically active, limiting alcoholic beverages, and following a heart-healthy eating plan.

In Summary

Hypertension remains a significant risk factor for general health and should not be ignored. Erectile dysfunction may be a very early warning sign for hypertension and for cardiovascular disease. One consistent theme throughout our discussion of the risk factors and treatments of erectile dysfunction is the importance of modifying the primary behavior, and such is also the case with hypertension.

If we don't modify primary risk factors, the disease process continues, and we merely manage the obvious symptoms with medication. Unfortunately, in the United States, we tend to treat risk factors separately without recognizing the underlying cause of the symptoms. Ask your doctor about proper blood pressure levels, appropriate therapies, and therapeutic lifestyle changes.

6

Low Testosterone and Sexual Dysfunction

Do you remember Woodstock? We mean the original concert in August 1969, not the copycats. If the answer is yes, then you are probably a baby boomer. It's been estimated that every single day, ten thousand people turn fifty. We are the baby boomers—220 million of us in midlife change.

As men become older, their bodies produce less testosterone, the male hormone that promotes the development and maintenance of male sex characteristics. Testosterone deficiency has been called the male menopause, the male change of life, or androgen deficiency in the aging male (ADAM).

How Testosterone Works

Testosterone is a member of the androgen family of hormones. Androgens include both testosterone and its metabolically active by-product called dihydrotestosterone, which is hormonally active in the prostate and related structures. Before birth, testosterone was required to create differentiation of the male sex organs, specifically the penis, scrotum, and prostate.

These same hormones are responsible for the start of sexual maturity. Testosterone is strongly related to sexual behavior and function, sperm production, and the development of male secondary sexual characteristics. These characteristics include male hair distribution on the chest, abdomen, and pubic area. Testosterone is also responsible for the male's deeper voice.

Testosterone is also required for the maintenance of muscle mass and the decrease of body fat, much like that you might see in an in-shape twenty-year-old man. Testosterone is also a necessary hormone for the development of the enzyme that is responsible for the production of nitric oxide, a cellular transmitter that is extremely important for the health of our arteries and endothelium.

Testosterone Levels Decrease with Age

We know that after the age of thirty, a man may lose up to 2 percent of testicular testosterone production each year. We also know that 20 to 50 percent of healthy men between the ages of fifty and seventy and even some at ages twenty to forty have lower than normal levels of testosterone. This suggests that up to 5 percent of all men are at risk for a low testosterone status. According to Census Bureau projections, the number of men in the United States between the ages of forty and fifty-five will be close to 60 million by the year 2020. This is a potentially large number of men with low testosterone.

Testosterone Decline Deficiency

When testosterone levels drop, our body fat levels increase, our muscle mass decreases, and we begin to develop the abdominal visceral fat that we discussed in chapter 2. Visceral fat is responsible for inflammatory and metabolic changes that can affect our bodies and put us at risk for cardiovascular disease. We also experience decreased bone mass, meaning our bones become more brittle. We have decreased sex drive and erectile dysfunction. We are also prone to depression and even decreased self-esteem.

Benefits of Testosterone Replacement Therapy

As their normal testosterone levels decrease with age, a growing number of healthy, older men are seeking testosterone replacement therapy. Testosterone therapy should be used only after careful evaluation by your physician. For many men, the therapy can be beneficial. Note that the much-publicized abuse of steroids by bodybuilders has nothing to do with the medically-supervised use of testosterone replacement therapy in men with low levels of testosterone.

Improved Sexual Function

A recent study found that after one week of therapy, men noticed improvement in sexual function and sexual motivation. By week four, erections began to improve. The response seen with testosterone therapy is durable. When the patients were examined at one year, they had improved measurements of their sexual functioning, including sexual motivation, sexual desire, improvement in spontaneous erections, and an increase in sexual intercourse. Many of them had also lost significant body fat and increased body muscle mass and bone mineral density.

Interestingly, several studies have addressed the optimal testosterone level to maximize erectile improvement; these levels typically range toward the higher end. Morning erections are directly correlated with testosterone levels; when the testosterone replacement is sufficient, morning erections return. We use the occurrence of morning erections almost as a clinical guide to determine whether a man's testosterone levels have increased.

Improved Mood

In some individuals, depression improved to the point that they did not need to continue taking antidepressants. However, any changes in medications such as antidepressants should only be undertaken after consulting your primary care physician.

Cardiovascular Benefits

Low testosterone levels are common in men with coronary artery disease and Type II Diabetes. Testosterone replacement therapy improves insulin sensitivity and glycemic control in men with diabetes and improves other cardiovascular risk factors.

We know that low testosterone levels affect heart health. Men who have had their testicles removed have been shown to be at greater risk for cardiovascular disease. Also, men who had long-term androgen deprivation therapy for prostate cancer had an increase in their insulin resistance, increasing their risk of cardiovascular disease.

Better Bone Density

Another significant risk factor seen with low testosterone is osteoporosis or brittle bones. When a man has a testosterone level less than 100 NG/DL, we believe it's an absolute indication to proceed with bone testing to rule out the presence of metabolic bone disorders. A stress fracture in a man, especially at a young age, should always prompt a workup for a low testosterone state. A particularly useful method to look for bone loss or osteoporosis in men is measuring height over time and comparing measurements with the loss of height seen with the aging process.

Other Benefits

Research shows that many men with diabetes also have low levels of testosterone. Testosterone has also been found to decrease insulin resistance in diabetic men. Low testosterone has also been linked to a number of clinical conditions, including the development of prostate cancer and Alzheimer's disease, as testosterone has been reported to have a positive effect on the memory and brain function.

How Is Testosterone Administered?

There are several new options available for testosterone replacement therapy for a man who needs it. In fact, the development of the testosterone gel has played a role in the growing popularity of this therapy.

Testosterone Gels

In the United States, the advent of testosterone gels, which are a convenient way to treat low testosterone, has revolutionized the treatment of testosterone deficiency. The gel, which is rubbed into the skin, is usually applied once a day, in the morning. Different brands of the gel are available, and application instructions vary among brands. Instructions with one brand may instruct you to rub the gel into your shoulders and upper arms; another brand may instruct you to rub the gel onto your abdomen. The gel should *never* be applied to the genitals.

It is important to use testosterone gel exactly as directed. Most men notice effects of the treatment within one to two weeks.

Testosterone Patches

Testosterone patches are called transdermal patches because they are applied to the skin and, like the gels, the testosterone preparation enters the body through the skin. Varying brands have different instructions for how to use the patches. One brand may instruct that a patch be applied at night and left on for twenty-four hours; another brand may instruct you to apply the patch in the morning and leave it in place for a day.

Some brands of patches are worn on the back, upper arm, thigh, or abdomen. One brand instructs you to apply the patch to your scrotum. It may take several weeks before you feel the full effect of the testosterone patch.

Gels and Patches Replace Injections

Before the topical testosterone therapies, the vast majority of men needing testosterone replacement were treated with testosterone injections. Testosterone was mixed with a vehicle such as cottonseed oil and injected deep into the muscle. The oil allowed the testosterone to be released slowly.

The downside to this treatment was that it required injections between one week and one month apart. These were often done in a physician's office, although, in some cases, the patient could self-inject after adequate training. Another drawback was the varying levels of testosterone that resulted. Testosterone levels went very high at the initial injection, creating an almost euphoric state. When the testosterone dropped below the normal levels, patients would often complain of depression and mood changes.

On a related note, there are newer testosterone preparations including a long-acting injectable testosterone medication, that lasts up to three months. This compound is widely available in Europe and is currently undergoing clinical trials in the United States.

Oral Testosterone

Oral testosterone preparations are also available. However, the preparations that are currently available in the United States are manufactured by a process that requires the liver to remove a certain part of the testosterone molecule to be metabolically active. This process in the liver is very toxic; this type of treatment regimen has a high incidence of liver problems and therefore is not recommended.

The only safe and effective oral testosterone preparation, a product called testosterone undeconoate, is expensive and requires multiple daily dosing to obtain a physiological level. It is available in Canada and elsewhere but not in the United States.

Evaluating Testosterone Levels

Before beginning testosterone therapy, a diagnostic workup is performed by your clinician. The diagnosis of testosterone deficiency is based both on symptoms reported by the patient and on the results of medical laboratory tests. We never treat patients who have an isolated laboratory finding of a low serum total testosterone without associated symptoms. In men who choose to proceed with testosterone therapy, close monitoring is very important.

Medical History

The patient's medical history will also determine cardiovascular health and whether a man may have diabetes; many men with Type II Diabetes have low testosterone levels as a consequence of the hormonal changes resulting from the diabetes. Other diagnostic clues to a low testosterone level include the loss of morning erections, depression, loss of muscle mass, and increased visceral body fat.

The medical history includes all the factors that are included in the ADAM (androgen deficiency in the aging male) questionnaire, which addresses erectile status, rigidity, and the ability to maintain the erection until completion of satisfactory sexual relations.

Prostate and Testicle Exam

A careful prostate examination is a must to assess the size and contour of the prostate and, most importantly, to rule out any prostate nodules, which can be a clue to the presence of prostate cancer. Testosterone is known to promote cancer growth, so it's important to determine that the prostate gland is healthy.

We also examine the testicles to assess their size and consistency to make sure that there are no testicular lesions that are interfering with testosterone production.

Androgen Deficiency in the Aging Male (ADAM) Questionnaire

1. Do you have a decrease in libido (sex drive)?
   Yes   No

2. Do you have a lack of energy?
   Yes   No

3. Do you have a decrease in strength and/or endurance?
   Yes   No

4. Have you lost height?
   Yes   No

5. Have you noticed a decreased enjoyment of life?
   Yes   No

6. Are you sad and/or grumpy?
   Yes   No

7. Are your erections less strong?
   Yes   No

8. During sexual intercourse, has it been more difficult to maintain your erection to completion of intercourse?
   Yes   No

9. Are you falling asleep after dinner?
   Yes   No

10. Has there been a recent deterioration in your work performance?
    Yes   No

If you answered YES to any of the above questions, you may have low testosterone levels. Fortunately there is something your doctor can do to help. Be sure to discuss the results of this questionnaire with your doctor.

Source: John E. Morley, MB, B.Ch, St. Louis University

Lab Tests

There are a number of laboratory tests that can be used to make the diagnosis of hypogonadism, or a low testosterone level. The most commonly available laboratory test checks levels of serum total testosterone, which is simply the amount of testosterone circulating in the blood. This is a widespread and inexpensive test, and is understood by most clinicians. Typically, normal testosterone levels range between 300 and 1,000 mg/dL. Young men tend to have higher levels, and as men age, the level tends to decrease.

Monitoring Men Using Testosterone Replacement

If testosterone replacement therapy is prescribed, it is crucial that your health practitioner perform routine blood tests during the course of therapy. In our practice, we draw blood to check testosterone levels after the first month of therapy; this helps us determine whether we need to adjust the dosage. Thereafter, we check levels every six months.

The monitoring of testosterone replacement therapy should be undertaken by a well-trained clinician dedicated to the observance of very strict parameters. These parameters have been well detailed and include measurement of the serum prostate specific antigen (PSA); a complete blood count (CBC), which is a group of blood tests; testosterone levels; and sometimes measurement of some of the breakdown products of testosterone such as estradiol. Estradiol is a dominant form of estrogen, the female hormone. In certain men, particularly those who have higher body levels of fat, the body may convert the testosterone to estradiol, affecting the man's levels of testosterone. In a small percentage of men, the estradiol can cause gynocomastia, an enlargement of the male breasts.

Checking Red Blood Cell Levels

When a man is on testosterone therapy, we monitor his red blood cell count. Why is this important? Testosterone preparations can raise the red blood cell count and create a condition known as polycythemia. This condition can cause the blood to become thick, raising the risk for stroke or heart attack. If it is determined that the red blood cell count is high, it may mean a lower dosage of testosterone is needed or it may mean the patient must discontinue the use of it for several weeks. At the end of this period, the red blood cell level can be checked again.

Checking PSA Levels

Total testosterone level should also be measured on a regular basis as a guide to the appropriate dose. If the prostate specific antigen (PSA) is elevated before the introduction of testosterone therapy, a prostate workup should be done by an experienced urologist. If the PSA remains elevated on a repeat blood test, a prostate ultrasound and possible prostate biopsy may be indicated depending on the treating urologist's clinical judgment. If the PSA is elevated the absence of prostate cancer must be confirmed prior to starting testosterone replacement.

A normal PSA level is not the same for everyone. It varies depending on age and ethnicity.

PSA Measurements

Age	Normal PSA	African American Normal PSA
40-50	2.5 or lower	2.0 or lower
50-60	3.5 or lower	3.0 or lower
60-70	4.5 or lower	4.0 or lower

Is Testosterone-Replacement Therapy Safe?

There is much new research on testosterone replacement therapy as it becomes more popular with the baby boomers and as we understand more about the significant positive effects of treatment. Although we see many improvements in a man's quality of life with testosterone replacement, there are potential side effects of the therapy. These include elevation of the cholesterol and red blood cell count, fluid retention, hepatitis, liver tumors, enlargement of the prostate, flare-up of preexisting prostate cancer, decreased testicle size, acne, infertility, mood swings, and high blood pressure.

Some members of the scientific and medical communities say large, long-term studies are needed on the effectiveness and safety of testosterone replacement therapy.

In Summary

Overall, testosterone plays a central role in the diagnosis and treatment of erectile dysfunction. There are newer testosterone replacement alternatives currently under study. We predict that testosterone replacement therapy will be essential to the maintenance of sexual health status and promoting cardiovascular care.

PART III

Diagnosis and Treatment for ED

7

How Erectile Dysfunction
Is Diagnosed

Recent studies have shown that up to 70 percent of
men with erectile dysfunction do not seek diagnosis
and treatment. There are many reasons for this. First,
when a man realizes that he has ED, it may lead to a range of
feelings, including: embarrassment, shame, failure, self-
doubt, shyness, inferiority, anxiety, depression, fear, appre-
hension, loneliness, disconnection with his partner and others, anger, resentment, and frustration. These are heavy,
destructive emotions, and they can take a toll on both the
physical and emotional intimacy in a man's life.

There are other reasons men do not seek treatment.
Some men are simply uninformed—they hold the common
belief that sexual dysfunction is part of the normal aging
process and an inevitable part of life. For some men, the cost
of treatment is an issue. Or perhaps the man and his partner
are not comfortable with the health care provider, and their
discomfort and embarrassment prevents them from pursuing
treatment.

However, there is good news: with today's diagnostic
tools and treatment options, there are many ways to overcome erectile dysfunction. It starts by finding a clinician you
trust.

Finding the Right Doctor

Finding the best physician to diagnose and treat erectile dysfunction is as important as finding the right doctor for any other health issue. Because of the intimacy of this problem, it's essential that you feel comfortable enough to share the most personal aspects of your life. Your doctor will explore your concerns from every angle, which means you'll be asked to share many personal details while also undergoing both a physical exam and a battery of tests. As a baby boomer with access to the Internet, you probably already have gathered a fair amount of information to get you started. Below are areas you'll want to concentrate on in your search.

Physician's Credentials

The best person to address your erectile dysfunction is a urologist, a physician who specializes in both male and female urinary tracts as well as male reproductive organs. Beyond medical school, these specialists complete at least five years of hands-on training in an accredited urology residency. In addition to exposure to general and urological surgery, urologists focus on many other topics, including sexual problems of both genders, particularly men's problems. Many urologists work in partnership with nurse practitioners and physician's assistants; you may see one of these healthcare professionals as part of your evaluation and treatment.

You may also need to consult a cardiologist who focuses on these issues for the obvious reason that there's a link between ED and the heart. Cardiologists, too, go through rigorous programs, but in their case the focus is on various problems of the heart.

In either case, you'll want to review this person's credentials to make sure that he or she has not only graduated from U.S.-accredited programs but also is certified (or candidate-ready) by the American Board of Urology (or the American College of Cardiology for cardiologists). What does that mean? Board certification indicates that in addition to fulfilling the educational and training requirements for licensure in the state, your doctor has undergone further testing and credentials review by his or her peers. It reflects a voluntary commitment to lifelong learning within the medical specialty.

You might also want to see how much this clinician is involved in professional organizations, attends clinical meetings, writes journal articles, or participates in clinical trials involving erectile dysfunction. Those activities also indicate a breadth of experience and willingness to keep up with the latest developments and newest treatments.

Seeking Referrals

But where do you find the names of qualified urologists? Your internist or family physician will likely give you an appropriate referral. But as with other health issues demanding the skills of a specialist, you can also look for the right match on your own. Ask friends or family members. Attend seminars on the subject. Or even peruse the Internet for the names of urologists who specialize in male sexual dysfunction.

A good place to start is with the American Board of Medical Specialties Web site, www.abms.org. Just click on "Consumers" and then "Find a Board Certified Specialist Here." If you don't have access to the information superhighway, you can also locate a copy of *The Official ABMS Directory* in most public and medical libraries. It gives biographical sketches of various board members.

Making the Most of Your Appointment

A resume can only tell you so much about someone's credentials to deal with your intimacy issues. The rest you'll need to discover from your first appointment. That's when you find out if you'll be comfortable enough with this person to describe the problem and follow his or her advice. Two good rules of thumb are to go prepared and trust your gut feeling.

The Internet has put medical information, including that concerning erectile dysfunction, at your fingertips. You can arm yourself with the basics of this topic in the privacy of your home, but here's the caveat: Be sure you're landing on reliable health sites. Web sites such as MedlinePlus (www.medlineplus.gov) and UrologyHealth (www.Urology Health.org) are good places to begin your search. The first is a consumer health resource linked to the National Library of Medicine. The American Urological Association Foundation sponsors the second site. Both offer accurate, even physician-reviewed material, on erectile dysfunction. By researching the topic in advance of your office visit, you can frame your thoughts and compose a list of questions to maximize your face-to-face meeting.

How you react to the physician in person and how he or she responds to you and your questions are an important factors in selecting treatment. Is the physician knowledgeable about the latest treatment options? Does he or she explain the choices in patient-speak so you understand what is being discussed? Do you have a good feeling about your interaction with this doctor and his or her interest in you? If you answer "no" to any of the above, you might want to move on. If, however, you have a good feeling from your first meeting, you may have found the perfect match.

Finally, if you're in a relationship while you're seeking help for your sexual dysfunction, make sure that your mate accompanies you to the appointment. Having your partner aware of the issues and familiar with the treatment can only benefit your relationship.

Your Medical History

Every evaluation for erectile and other sexual dysfunctions begins with a detailed health history and physical examination. Since age is one of the greatest risk factors for these problems, your doctor will begin with that basic. From there, he or she will explore many aspects of your personal and family health history.

Since sexual dysfunction can be an early sign of more-serious cardiovascular issues, your doctor will be interested in all matters related to your heart. He or she will want to know if you have a history of coronary artery disease or symptoms related to other cardiac issues. You'll be asked about many related topics, including your family history of diabetes and your own exercise and dietary habits.

Knowing that you eat foods rich in saturated fat and trans-fatty acids, as well as carbohydrates and processed items, is an important diagnostic clue for erectile dysfunction since such dietary choices facilitate inflammation of the arteries, including those to the genitalia. Similarly, your doctor will want to know about the amount of routine exercise you get. Exercising (or not exercising) can have an effect on sexual function. (We suggest a thirty-minute cardiovascular workout on most days in addition to weight training three days a week. If that's not possible, a minimum of three twenty-minute episodes per week is a good goal.)

Because tobacco is known to constrict the blood vessels, while contributing to a host of cardiac and other health problems, your physician will want to know your smoking habits. Don't be surprised if the doctor focuses on the type of tobacco in addition to the number of years you've smoked. Marijuana, for instance, can expose you to the same tobacco-related risks as cigarettes, so it's important to share that information.

Sexual Function

Your physician must explore every aspect of your sexual function to get to the root of the problem. So be prepared to answer very intimate questions about the timing, duration, and quality of your erections as well as your general experience with intercourse. He or she will want to know, for instance, about your ability to achieve an erection with or without appropriate sexual stimulation as well as your ability to maintain it during sexual activity. Although the average interval between penetration and ejaculation is about two and a half minutes, the length of intercourse won't be as significant to your doctor. He or she will be focused on your ability to maintain the erection and achieve ejaculation, not on how long it takes you to do so.

Since many conditions can prevent you from normal ejaculation or can lead to retrograde ejaculation, taking your medical history will be paramount. Your doctor will be concerned about priapism, a painful and prolonged erection that can last for several hours or days. Although the causes of this condition are poorly understood, research points to a complex set of vascular and neurological issues as well as some medications. Penile injections to achieve erections in the first place are often the culprit.

Your doctor may use either the International Index of Erectile Dysfunction (IIEF) or a shortened version, the Sexual Health Inventory in Men (SHIM), to determine the frequency and quality of your erections. These quick questionnaires (see Appendix) are important diagnostic tools in evaluating your issues.

Medication Review

Since erectile dysfunction can be caused by certain medications, it's important to document all of your prescription and nonprescription drugs for the doctor. Many commonly used agents can affect a man's ability to achieve and maintain an erection. You may already be familiar with some of them: Beta-blockers and thiazide diuretics, for instance, are very effective in treating high blood pressure and some post–heart attack health issues, but they also can cause or worsen sexual dysfunction. Similarly, selective serotonin reuptake inhibitors (SSRIs) are widely tolerated medications for depression, but they can also inhibit a man's ability to produce a quality ejaculation. In your listing, you'll also want to include any samples of erectile dysfunction agents, such as Viagra, Levitra, or Cialis, that you might have received from another physician or friend to correct the problem.

Since herbal and other over-the-counter remedies can also affect your sexual function, you need to document those medicines as well. In fact, some of the herbs used to improve erectile function actually contain adulterated quantities of sildenafil, the generic form of Viagra. Other over-the-counter remedies may cause genitourinary irritations, which can trigger negative results. Moreover, many weight-loss products and sinus medicines contain a compound called ephedra, which can lessen the quality of an erection. Men with chronic sinusitis, sinus drainage, or allergies who take nonprescription decongestants, for instance, often have poor performance.

Since your physician needs a complete medicinal picture to make a correct diagnosis, take the time to be thorough in compiling your list before your office visit.

Physical Examination

After your physician completes a patient history, he or she will focus on the physical examination. It's important for the doctor to evaluate your genitalia to see if there are physical reasons for your erectile dysfunction. He or she will examine many parts of your anatomy in great detail.

Testicles (Testes)

Because the size of your testicles correlates directly with the amount of male hormone, or testosterone, that you produce, your doctor will focus on their dimension and texture during the exam. If your testes were damaged at some point in your life (for example from teenage mumps), the size might have been diminished, which can have a dramatic effect on your testosterone production.

65

Scrotum (Scrotal Sac)

Because the scrotum, the sac that contains your testicles, can have a bearing on your testes, your doctor will examine it closely. He or she will be looking for any evidence of a varicocele, a varicose vein–like enlargement of the vessels in your scrotum. Commonly occurring on the left side, a varicocele can adversely affect testicular size as well as the volume and quality of sperm. The good news is that varicoceles can be surgically repaired.

Penis

By examining your penis, your doctor can rule out various conditions that can be inhibiting your sexual function. The physician can see, for instance, if you have Peyronie's disease, a scarring of tissue on the organ that can cause it to bend when erect. In some cases, the Peyronie's bow is so profound that it makes intercourse impossible.

The doctor also checks for decreased blood flow, referred to as arterial dysfunction, into the penis. That's important because this organ, like any other in your body, needs sufficient blood flow to perform adequately. During the exam, your doctor will palpate the arterial pulses in your groin and the pedal pulses in your feet. Combined, the two measures give a rough diagnostic estimate of blood flow to the lower extremities. An absence of pulses in your feet, accompanied by coolness and decreased hair on your lower extremities, indicates poor blood flow.

Before we leave this topic, let us clarify a common myth about penis length. It isn't usually related to erectile function (or dysfunction), even though a longer penis can be important cosmetically for some men. Many factors can cause your penis to shrink, including prior surgical procedures for prostate cancer and Peyronie's disease. You also can expect the loss of penile length as you move into mid and later life. Your penis won't be the same size at age fifty, sixty, or seventy as it was at twenty. Also, for every thirty-five pounds of weight gain, according to one estimate, the penis appears to lose one inch of length.

Prostate

Your physician will perform a digital exam to determine the health of your prostate. Although inserting a gloved finger into the rectum may cause momentary discomfort, it's a simple way to test if the prostate is either enlarged or has nodules associated with prostate cancer. With the digital exam, your doctor can also check for other lesions in the rectum that may be symptoms of colorectal cancer.

Laboratory Tests

Your physician can't make an accurate diagnosis without conducting several laboratory and other tests. The good news is that many technological and testing modalities exist today to help your physician assess both your general and sexual health. He or she will rely on several lab tests, starting with those below.

Urinalysis

A urinalysis can help your physician identify potential underlying causes of erectile dysfunction. It yields a wealth of information on protein, sugar, and testosterone levels. Abnormal measures can indicate diabetes, kidney disease, or testosterone deficiencies, all of which can trigger erectile dysfunction. Glucose and/or microscopic albumin protein (a condition known as microalbuminuria) are both diagnostic indicators for diabetes. The presence of albumin protein also indicates hypertension and endothelial dysfunction, an independent risk factor for cardiovascular disease in addition to a strong indicator of erectile dysfunction.

Complete Blood Count (CBC)

A complete blood count can reveal much about the state of your overall and sexual health. A measure of white and red cells along with other blood components, a CBC can detect problems such as anemia. Caused by low red cells, anemia can trigger fatigue, which, in turn, contributes to erectile dysfunction.

Fasting Glucose

By measuring the amount of sugar in the blood, this test offers a simple way to diagnose or screen for diabetes, one of the significant underlying causes of erectile dysfunction.

Lipid Profile

Lipid profiles are essential in tracking the level of fats, such as cholesterol, in your coronary arteries. Measuring low-density lipids (the "bad" cholesterol), high-density lipids (the "good" cholesterol), and triglycerides can help determine if you have hardening of the arteries, or atherosclerosis, which can decrease blood circulation to all of your organs, including your penis.

Homocysteine and C-reactive Protein Levels

Your doctor may also want to measure the levels of your homocysteines and C-reactive protein, two lesser-known but very important new markers of cardiovascular problems. Both facilitate blocked arteries. Homocysteines are amino acids used by the body in cellular metabolism. Elevated blood concentrations of homocysteines are believed to increase the risk for heart disease by damaging the lining of the vessels and enhancing clotting.

The liver produces C-reactive protein to respond when the body experiences inflammation, infection, or injury. When the irritation occurs in the lining of the blood vessels, it's linked to obesity, diabetes, and cardiovascular disease. By measuring the inflammation, a simple test called the C-reactive protein test has given doctors an excellent tool to predict future cardiovascular events. In the case of the heart, elevated protein levels indicate inflammation in the endothelial or lining tissues. That indicates an increased risk for cardiovascular problems, which could affect your penis.

Prolactin

The hormone prolactin is emitted by the pituitary gland, and elevated levels of serum prolactin in the blood can indicate various health issues including impotence. Some medications also can increase the normal range of production, which falls between 2 and 18 ng/ml (nanograms per milliliter) in men.

Testosterone Levels

Used to diagnose sexual-related conditions in both men and women, a testosterone analysis is routinely ordered if a patient complains of decreased sex drive or erectile dysfunction. A common occurrence as men age, lower

Paul's Story

How important is a cardiovascular workup? Consider Paul F., a forty-three-year-old patient with a history of inability to achieve and maintain erections. He was referred to us for evaluation after trying unsuccessfully to correct the problem with Viagra. By discussing his medical history, we discovered that Paul was a heavy smoker who had multiple risk factors for cardiovascular disease, including a family history of diabetes.

By running a variety of tests, we were able to complete a fairly detailed picture of our patient, who was at risk for coronary problems. Paul's urinalysis was positive for glucose and microalbuminuria, a marker for endothelial dysfunction. His ultrasound demonstrated poor blood flow and a significant vessel leak. Given his risk factors, and an off-the-cuff mention of chest pains at work, we made an immediate referral to a cardiologist. Before he knew it, Paul had to undergo a heart catheterization and have two stents inserted. He came to us about his ED, but the visit probably saved his life.

testosterone can affect sexual characteristics such as facial and body hair, voice depth, and muscle development. But it also can indicate myriad issues, including damage to the testes and other diseases. Your physician will use this test to identify any underlying problems. Because reference standards are dependent on many factors, including your age and a specific lab's numeric values, there's no one standard range. Your physician can make sense of the numbers as they pertain to you.

Prostate-Specific Antigen (PSA)

A simple blood test for prostate cancer, the PSA test is based on the presence of a protein, prostate-specific antigen, produced by the prostate gland. High levels of PSA may indicate the presence of a cancerous tumor, although other health issues, such as prostatitis (inflammation of the prostate) and benign prostatic hyperplasia (enlargement of the gland), can also be at fault. Although your doctor will likely order this test to rule out a malignancy, it may also yield information about other issues underlying your ED.

Other Tests to Help in Diagnosis

Physicians rely on more than just laboratory tests to diagnose erectile dysfunction. Because of today's sophisticated imaging and other technology, they can accurately evaluate a man's sexual function. Your doctor will likely call for additional tests. Here's just a sampling.

Nocturnal Penile Tumescence (NPT)

By measuring a man's erectile function during sleep, this test provides a baseline look at a patient's sexual function as well as other potential issues. How so? Men normally have five or six erections during sleep. A lesser number of them can indicate issues with nerve function or circulation in the penis.

The RigiScan Plus Rigidity Assessment System exemplifies the "strain gauge method" of measuring NPT. It works by placing loops of wire strain gauge material over the penis to record the quality and duration of nighttime erections. When the penis becomes erect, the material stretches, gauging changes in its circumference. A second or "snap gauge method" involves wrapping three plastic bands of varying length around the penis. Erectile function is measured based on which band breaks.

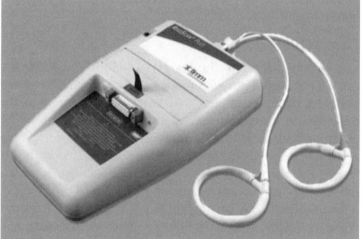

Photo Courtesy of Timm Medical, Eden Prairie, MN

The RigiScan measures the rigidity of a man's erections overnight. The test can be done at home; a man places the loops around his penis before going to sleep.

Penile Doppler Ultrasound

A real-time color-flow ultrasound of the penis is probably the most valuable test physicians have in identifying the causes of erectile dysfunction. Doppler ultrasounds use high-frequency sound waves to snap pictures of the body's internal tissues. In men with suspected ED, they're used to evaluate blood flow and check for signs of underlying health issues such as tissue scarring or atherosclerosis. After injecting a vasoactive medication into the penis to stimulate an erection, the doctor proceeds with an ultrasound examination.

The test may also involve examining the penis when it's flaccid, or soft. The results can yield precise information about many issues, including blood flow, potential vascular leaks, and the presence of Peyronie's plaques. An ultrasound is particularly useful in men with a long history of uncontrolled diabetes who haven't been responsive to conservative treatments for their ED. It's also used prior to any corrective surgery. In any case, this test offers a very helpful glimpse into the potential causes of erectile dysfunction.

Exercise Stress Test

Sometimes referred to as a treadmill test, a stress test can help your doctor determine just how well your heart performs during exercise. We know that every time the body has to exert more effort, the heart must respond by pumping additional blood. But how good is it at doing that? A stress test reveals if the blood supply is reduced in the arteries supplying the heart during exercise. Performed under the watchful eye of a primary care physician or cardiologist, it involves walking on the treadmill at graduated speeds while being monitored by various cardio-monitoring machines. That includes an electrocardiogram (ECG or EKG), which records the electrical activity of the heart.

If your physician suspects any heart health issues because of your medical history, severely abnormal cholesterol or lipid profiles, or other risk factors, he or she will likely order a stress test. Depending on the results, you may need a further cardiac workup.

Endothelial Testing

Although testing for endothelial function/dysfunction in patients with erectile problems has evolved, it still isn't part of mainstream practice. Your physician is unlikely to order it since this type of testing is performed at large research centers and is not covered by most insurance policies.

In Summary

Your physician may determine that other tests are necessary. The point is, with the right doctor and a willingness to be open about your symptoms, you can get to the root of your sexual problems. Urologists as well as other doctors see many men who have taken the first steps toward a satisfactory sex life by recognizing the problem and seeking expert advice. As you'll learn in the next chapter, your doctor can choose from many treatment options.

8

Treatment for Erectile Dysfunction

The medical treatments for sexual dysfunction have undergone many changes in the past two decades. In years past, we commonly thought that most men with sexual dysfunction had a psychological problem and that counseling was the most important therapy. Now, we know that the primary problem for sexual dysfunction in men is often not psychological, but rather, the "equipment failure" is related to physical impairments, most often to decreased blood flow.

Medications for ED

We mentioned earlier that the 1998 release of the first erectile dysfunction drug started a new sexual revolution. To date, ED drugs have been among the most-advertised products in the history of the United States, with nearly $8 billion spent annually on marketing. It seems we cannot watch a sporting event without seeing at least one ad for one of the PDE-5 inhibitors, such as Viagra.

No doubt, many men have achieved good results with the PDE-5 inhibitors. We began prescribing these drugs years ago and still prescribe them today. We usually start patients on one of the PDE-5 inhibitors—Viagra, Levitra, or Cialis—usually at higher doses, unless they are using nitroglycerin or alpha-blockers for heart conditions. As stressed earlier, combining the ED drugs with these heart medications can create blood pressure problems.

Finding the Right Medication

When we prescribe ED medications, we try each of them, Viagra, Cialis, and Levitra, one at a time, and we then work through our patient's responses and make appropriate changes based on the results. We want to use the medication that produces the best erection, has the longest duration, and has the fewest side effects. We think it's extremely important that men have multiple opportunities to try each of these medications. Several studies have shown that when a man does not respond to treatment with a PDE-5 inhibitor, generally it either was not dosed properly or not dosed long enough.

Most of the drug studies for the approval of the PDE-5 inhibitors were done in men who had mild to moderate sexual dysfunction, not the group of "hard-to-treat" men. For example, men with prostate cancer who have had various surgical treatments or men who have significant diabetes, hypertension, and various medications related to this may need different doses, different drug options, or longer periods of treatment before they will see results.

Getting the Dosage Right

When we prescribe ED drugs, we give patients meticulous dosing instructions. Several studies have shown that the success rate of PDE-5 inhibitors is dramatically improved when patients are given tailored instructions, rather than just handed sample packages of medication. This is especially true for patients with diabetes.

The different PDE-5 inhibitors require slightly different patient education and instruction. The PDE-5 inhibitors all inhibit the same enzyme but there are several nuances that make each one unique in clinical situations.

Viagra should be taken on an empty stomach without alcohol. It takes about an hour for the drug to start working, and it has a half-life of about four hours, meaning the drug stays in the body for four hours. If a man tells us he has not had a successful response to Viagra, we recommend that he take it daily for several days before attempting intercourse again. This can frequently lead to success for a substantial number of these patients.

Levitra can be taken with or without food and with or without alcohol and becomes effective in about one hour; it has a half-life of approximately four to five hours.

Cialis is taken daily and can be taken with or without food. It takes a little longer to start working—about an hour and a half to two hours—but can stay effective in the body for up to thirty-six hours. This length of time is dependent on the patient, how the patient metabolizes the medication, and, more importantly, the degree of sexual dysfunction. The FDA has approved daily dosing of Cialis, giving a man improved sexual response and a greater degree of choice in choosing when to be sexually active.

Medication Side Effects

The ED medications all have similar side effects, including headache, indigestion, flushing, and stuffy nose. One of the potential side effects of Viagra is sensitivity to light; also, some men have reported "blue vision," in which they see bluish tinges or have trouble distinguishing between green and blue. This side effect is usually seen only at very high doses and dissipates within a few hours.

Additionally, there has been press coverage linking these drugs to a low incidence of vision loss called nonarteritic anterior ischemic optic neuropathy (NAION). This form of vision loss occurs suddenly when blood flow to the optic nerve is blocked. However, research data has not justified this connection, and it is probably not of concern clinically. We often tell patients that if they notice a sudden change in their vision with these medications, they should stop taking them immediately and tell their doctor. We do not feel, however, that these medications are unsafe.

Cialis has a unique and infrequent side effect of muscle aches and back pains.

If chest pain occurs while taking any of the ED medications, you must tell the emergency room doctor that you have used these medications, because they can interact with the nitrates commonly used to treat patients with chest pain, causing life-threatening low blood pressure. As we mentioned earlier, do not take Viagra, Levitra, or Cialis with the drugs known as alpha-blockers or with nitroglycerin or amyl nitrate.

Include Your Partner in Discussing Medications

We engage both the man and his partner in a discussion of the treatment, answering questions about expectations and possible results. We teach our patients that these medications are not going to cure the cause of erectile dysfunction, but they are treating a symptom of ED. We also explain that even though the drugs help produce an erection, they do not increase arousal. Nor do they prevent pregnancy or protect against sexually transmitted diseases. If the patient's spouse or partner is not present for the visit, we encourage the man to talk to his partner about starting this medication.

Lifestyle Changes

Although these drugs help many men remain sexually active, one of the key factors in staying sexually active is leading a healthful lifestyle. Since the advent of these medications in 1998, it's not uncommon to see men who come to our office because these medications have stopped working for them. They may have started the medication in 1998 at low doses and slowly over the years have progressed to the highest dose, but it has become ineffective. This is because they have not changed their lifestyle and their primary risk factors, such as heart disease or high blood pressure, have not changed. We cannot emphasize enough that the ED drugs alone are not a cure for erectile dysfunction.

Herbal Preparations for ED

It's interesting that more men choose herbal remedies than use standard PDE-5 therapy for the treatment of erectile dysfunction. According to the American Urological Association, there are several herbs (see list below) that are used to treat ED. However, scientific proof of their effectiveness has not been established.

- **Asian ginseng** *(Panax ginseng):* Traditionally used for male impotence, though no current studies support this usage.
- **Damiana** *(Turnera diffusa):* Traditionally used as an aphrodisiac and for various sexual disorders; however, there are no current studies to confirm its effectiveness.
- **Ginkgo biloba**: Increases arterial blood flow, which may have a positive effect on male sexual function.
- **Muira puama** *(Ptychopetalum olacoides):* Used for erectile dysfunction and lack of libido.

Many men choose to purchase their herbs as well as medications on the Internet; it is important to make such purchases only from reputable sources. Otherwise, taking these drugs can be dangerous because it's impossible to know whether you're getting a quality preparation or one that's nonstandard, unpurified, or even toxic or poisonous.

Penile Injections

Another treatment option is penile injections, which have been available since the mid-1970s. A small, 30-gauge needle is used, the same type diabetics use for insulin injections. A man gives himself the injection, which is quite painless. Ejaculation sensations are preserved with this method.

Papaverine and Phentolamine

A drug commonly used for penile injection for ED is papaverine, which is mixed with a drug called phentolamine.

Papaverine was originally marketed for use in vascular surgery to dilate blood vessels. It was also taken as an oral medication to act

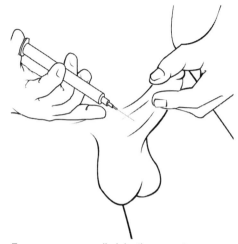

For some men, penile injections create an erection. The injections are relatively painless and contain drugs that enhance blood flow into the penis.

as a vasodilator in people with muscle pain, caused by lack of blood flow to the lower extremities and in people with vascular disease in the legs. Phentolamine is also a drug that causes blood vessels to expand.

Both of these drugs have been approved by the Food and Drug Administration; however, they were not officially approved for erectile dysfunction. This means they, like many drugs, were considered "off-label use" for ED. Still, the use of this drug combination for erectile dysfunction was so widespread throughout the 1980s that more of it was sold in its first year of use for ED than was sold in the previous thirty years.

Alprostadil

The drug alprostadil is effective as an injectable to help men achieve erections. The drug causes relaxation in the corporal smooth muscle, helping to produce an erection. The drug is well tolerated by most men. This product, now marketed as Caverject and Edex, comes in a dry powder form, and liquid is then added to it at the time of use in a self-dosing syringe. The drug is considered fast-acting and works for thirty to sixty minutes.

There are several other medications that can be mixed as injectables for men who have a poor response to the FDA-approved standard dosage regimens. Although each of these other medications is FDA-approved for other uses, their use for erectile dysfunction is considered "off-label." It's important to notify patients that these drugs are being used off-label. We generally use the more-exotic mixtures for patients for whom the standard regimens have failed.

Injection Side Effects

The most common side effect of these medications is burning. However, the burning is well controlled with combination mixtures of medications. The only other major concern is the side effect of a prolonged erection. This condition, also known as priapism, is defined as an erection that lasts more than four hours and is painful.

This side effect is somewhat common in men who use injections at much higher than recommended doses. We counsel these patients very carefully and use various medications such as *Sudafed*, or pseudoephedrine, to prevent this condition. We recommend that the patient use only one injection per day, no more than three to five times a week.

A note for men with diabetes: Penile injections are extremely useful and popular in men with diabetes, although these men frequently need higher doses with adjustments. The learning curve for teaching a man with diabetes to do penile injections is quick because many of these men are comfortable with a subcutaneous injection of insulin and the techniques are similar. The biggest risk for this method in the man with diabetes is infection. As long as patients use proper techniques and maintain tight glycemic control, the infection rate is close to zero percent.

Intraurethral Suppositories

The drug Alprostadil, which is the medication used for penile injections, is also used in intraurethral suppositories, which are marketed as *Muse* (medicated urethral suppository for erection). A man inserts this small pellet into his urethra at the tip of the penis and massages it until it dissolves.

This medication can produce an erection in a number of men but there are some drawbacks to its use. First, it may cause irritation and burning. Secondly, it's not as effective as a penile injection. And, finally, it's not as cost-effective as the injectable drug.

Prior to the newer ED drugs, intraurethral medications were popular in the 1990s, and there is still a loyal following of men who are very happy with Muse therapy. If this treatment works for you, it is certainly a reasonable choice.

Vacuum Devices

Other treatment options include the vacuum erection device (VED). This is not a new concept; it has been around for many years. A vacuum pump is a clear plastic cylinder that fits over the penis. Negative pressure is applied, and blood is pulled into the penis. A rubber ring placed at the base of the penis traps the blood and prevents it from escaping. The advantage to this device is that it is noninvasive and

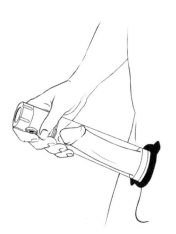

The vacuum device is a plastic tube that fits over the penis. As air is pumped out, blood is pulled into the penis, creating an erection.

81

relatively simple to use. The downside is that a VED produces a fairly swollen penis that tends to be cool to the touch, and you may have some loss of sensation.

Before the advent of modern vacuum erection devices, the majority of these devices were sold from the back of men's magazines as "penis enlargers." Clinicians tended to avoid them because they were not familiar with the devices and because there was little peer-reviewed medical literature on them. It wasn't until the National Institutes of Health Consensus Statement on Impotence (1992) that VEDs became a reasonable option in the treatment of erectile dysfunction. Vacuum erection devices, like many other devices, differ in quality. The adage "You get what you pay for" is true in choosing a VED.

Vacuum devices are not very popular among men with diabetes; the constriction ring can decrease sensation in the penis. This, coupled with the decreased sensation within the penis related to the diabetic neuropathy, can lead to a decrease in sexual pleasure.

ACTIS Ring

The ACTIS Ring, also known as a constriction ring, is a device intended to strengthen erections by slowing the flow of blood away from the penis. The ACTIS device consists of an adjustable loop that is placed around the base of the penis. An O-ring and ball-locking unit allow for easy adjustment of tension.

The device should not be worn longer than thirty minutes; wearing it longer could cause damage to penis tissues. You should allow sixty minutes between uses.

Penile Implants

Penile implants, or prostheses, are another alternative for men with erectile dysfunction. In the right patient, a penile implant is a blessing; however, in a poorly selected patient, it can be a nightmare.

Deciding to have a penile implant is a very important decision for a man, and there are many factors that need to be considered by both the patient and the implanting surgeon. Penile implant surgery is covered in depth in chapter 9.

Reconstructive Surgical Procedures

Vascular Surgical Procedures

There are two reconstructive surgical procedures for ED, but they are not commonly recommended. Vascular reconstructive surgery is performed to improve the blood supply to the penis in efforts to restore a man's ability to get and maintain an erection. The procedure is technically difficult and not always effective. Accordingly, it is rarely performed.

Vascular reconstructive surgery of the penis is very much like a coronary artery bypass graft except it's performed on the penis. It involves bypassing blocked arteries by transferring an artery from an abdominal muscle to a penile artery so that there is sufficient blood flow to the penis.

Another type of vascular reconstructive surgery is correction of venous leakage. As we described earlier, when the penis becomes erect, it fills with blood and veins close to trap the blood in order to maintain the erection. If the veins do not close well, blood leaks out. This is called a venous leak.

Vascular surgeries in the penis work only in a very select few patients, who are typically younger men with excellent blood flow who have had a dramatic injury to the penis or the perineum, the space between the scrotum and the rectum. These surgeries have never been perfected to the extent that they are reproducible and reliable in all cases and, therefore, have never really entered the mainstream except in methods of management of ED. The effectiveness of these types of surgeries is minimal at best.

The Costs of Treatment for ED

The financial responsibility for ED treatment plays a role in many men's adherence to a treatment program. The cost of the medication can be as much as $17 per pill; testosterone replacement can cost as much as $300 per month. The insurance reimbursement may be minimal or nonexistent. Some insurance companies view ED as a "quality of life" issue and do not cover treatment of any kind, no matter the cause. The cost of a visit to a health care professional, the diagnostic studies, and the prescribed treatment must all be considered.

In Summary

Treatment for erectile dysfunction needs to be individualized. The best solution for one person may not be the best for another. It's important to determine what each patient's goals are. Find a doctor with whom you are comfortable, and use the device or medication that produces an adequate erection for penetration. Always remember that many options are available.

9

Penile Implant Surgery

When medications, vacuum devices, or penile injections are not effective, or, more importantly, unsatisfactory for the treatment of erectile dysfunction, there are surgical options. The most-popular surgical option for ED is the penile implant. Penile implants have been around since the 1970s and were the first surgical treatments for erectile dysfunction. Since then, research in biomaterials has resulted in dramatically improved implant devices.

There are currently two categories of penile implants: malleable implants, sometimes called semi-rigid implants, and inflatable implants.

Malleable Implants

The malleable implant is a flexible device, made of silicone elastomer, a rubber-like material. It creates an erection that may be bent into position for sexual function. Some semi-rigid penile implants are more flexible than others, based on how they are made. Flexibility is a preference of some patients.

The malleable implant consists of two rods of varying flexibility. They are implanted into the corpora cavernosal bodies of the penis and provide an erection to facilitate sex-

Malleable Penile Implant

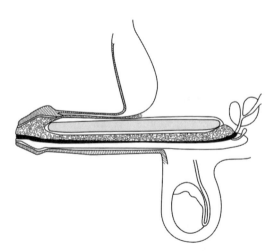

The malleable implant, pictured at the top, shows how the implant is bent straight for an erection. The bottom photo shows how the device is bent downward when a man does not wish to have an erection.

A malleable implant is straightened to create an erect penis.

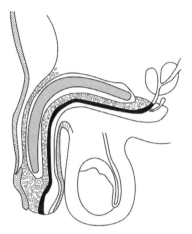

When not in use, the semi-rigid, or malleable, implant is bent downward manually.

Two-Piece Inflatable Implant

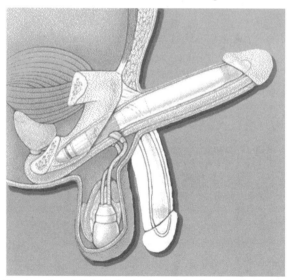

The two-piece inflatable implant consists of a pair of cylinders, which are placed in the penis, and a single pump, which is implanted in the scrotum.

Three-Piece Inflatable Implant

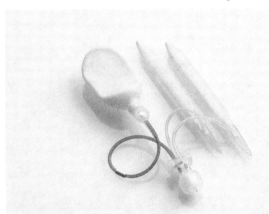

This three-piece inflatable implant consists of two cylinders, a reservoir that holds sterile saline, a pump that transfers the fluid to the cylinders, and touch-pads, used to deflate the implant.

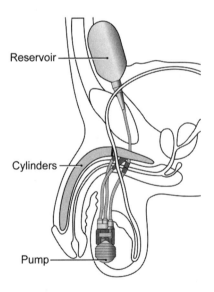

With a three-piece implant, two cylinders are inserted in the shaft of the penis. The reservoir is implanted in the lower abdomen, and the pump is placed in the scrotum.

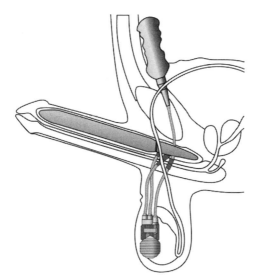

When a man wishes to have an erection, he manually turns on the pump in the scrotum, and fluid from the reservoir inflates the two cylinders.

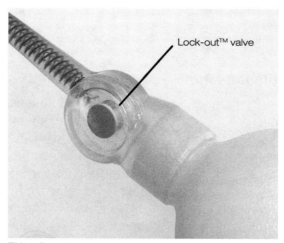

Lock-out™ valve

This inflatable implant has a lock-out valve, which prevents the implant from inflating or deflating accidentally.

ual penetration and intercourse. They work like bendable rods. These rods are bent upward for sexual activity and downward when not in use. The advantages of this type of penile implant are ease of placement and the need for minimum manipulation for usage. The disadvantage is that the penis has the appearance of always being partially erect.

In some European countries, the malleable penile implant is preferred as the implant of choice. In our practice, we have found that patients who have had a three-piece inflatable penile implant (see below) almost always are unhappy if they switch to a malleable penile implant.

The malleable penile implant is commonly used for a patient with a concealed penis, one that is no longer visible to the eye due to surrounding fat tissue. Other candidates for this type of implant are men who have decreased motor function in their hands and are unable to manipulate a penile inflation pump.

> The first attempt at a penile implant was performed in 1936 by a surgeon who implanted a piece of rib cartilage under the skin of a man's penis as a method to give him an erection adequate for penetration.

Inflatable Implants

In 1973, Brantley Scott, M.D., implanted the first inflatable penile prosthesis. Since then, the reliability of the device has been improved dramatically, and the inflatable penile implant has evolved into the gold standard of penile implants. The inflatable penile implant has two categories: the two-piece implant and the three-piece implant.

The two-piece device consists of two cylinders with a bulb, which serves as a combined reservoir and pump mechanism; this bulb is placed in the scrotum. When a man desires an erection, he squeezes the pump, and fluid transfers to the cylinders, creating an erection. When a man wishes to deflate the implant, he bends it down for six to twelve seconds and then releases it; this causes the reservoir to open and the fluid flows out of the cylinders.

This type of implant has the appearance of always being partially erect and does not provide the natural appearance of the three-piece devices; nor does it provide the same rigidity or flaccidity that can be achieved with the three-piece implant.

The three-piece inflatable implant, which is the main focus of this chapter, is essentially a hydraulic system consisting of a reservoir, two cylinders, and a pumping device. The reservoir holds the fluid, which is typically sterile saline solution. The two cylinders are implanted within the corporal bodies of the penis. The pump, which transfers the fluid, is implanted in the scrotal sac. To get an erection, a man squeezes the pump a few times, causing the fluid to fill the cylinders. To make the penis return to a flaccid state, a man continuously squeezes the release bars attached to the reservoir, and the implant deflates.

Choosing an Implant

The decision as to which penile implant to choose should be made by the patient and his surgeon, who will consider the patient's health and manual strength and dexterity. The most popular implant in the United States, the three-piece implant gives the most-natural-looking penis both when erect and nonerect. Given the popularity, reliability, and availability of the three-piece device, we seldom recommend the malleable implants to our patients.

Benefits of a Penile Implant

The penile prosthesis is considered to be the permanent surgical treatment for erectile dysfunction. Worldwide, more than 26,000 men receive penile implants each year. (Ten times that number of breast implant procedures are performed in the U.S. annually.) The surgical implantation of the inflatable penile implant provides these positive results:

- Reliable and predictable erections
- Natural appearance of the erection
- Implant is hidden within the body
- Penis has a more-natural, youthful appearance when deflated
- Easy-to-use pumping device, making erections almost instantaneous and spontaneous
- Long-term solution to erectile dysfunction
- Ability to maintain the erection as long as needed
- No further recurring cost involved for pills or injections
- Short outpatient surgical time, resulting in low surgical risk
- Custom-fitted to the body
- High rate of patient and partner satisfaction
- Short recovery time
- Covered by most insurance companies

High Satisfaction Rates

Today, the penile implant is associated with a high rate of satisfaction among men and their partners. When a skilled surgeon performs penile implant surgery, the results show a patient satisfaction rate that exceeds 95 percent in most cases. Partner satisfaction is greater than 90 percent. An erection can be achieved on demand and can be maintained for as long as needed. Further, the implant does not constrict or interfere with ejaculatory ducts, so it does not interfere with a man's ability to ejaculate. These advantages allow men to confidently put spontaneity back into their sexual relationship. If an unexpected interruption occurs during sexual activity, the inflatable implant is easily deflated and can be inflated at a more-convenient time.

Preoperative Evaluation

The preoperative evaluation of erectile function and dysfunction should be determined by careful physical examination. During this examination, the surgeon will determine the presence or absence of penile scarring such as seen with Peyronie's disease; the surgeon will also predict the length of the cylinders that will be placed into the penis during the surgery. This measurement is done by traction on the penis and will give an accurate representation of the penile length that will be obtained after implantation of the device.

Additional considerations in the preoperative evaluation include a determination of blood flow to the penis. In our practice, we utilize the color-flow penile Doppler ultrasound test, which we described in chapter 7. During this test, a medication, such as prostaglandin, which produces a maximum erection with sexual stimulation, is injected into the penis. Blood flow is measured at the peak of the erection.

The ultrasound will determine the degree of blood flow to and from the penis as well as determine the presence or absence of Peyronie's disease. It is also helpful in determining the best method of treatment for ED. If the patient responds favorably to the penile injection and achieves a rigid erection, we may recommend that the man use injection therapy rather than receive a penile implant.

The status of the scrotum is examined at the time of the workup as another critical part of the preoperative evaluation. The implant pumping mechanism will be placed within the scrotal sac, so it is important to determine the presence or absence of scarring and the location of the testes. At this time, the doctor also exams the lower abdomen and pelvis for various scars and hernias. This enables the surgeon to determine the best surgical approach for the placement of the penile implant and placement of the reservoir.

Surgical Implant Procedure

The surgery may be performed in an inpatient or outpatient setting. Anesthesia may be light sedation or general anesthesia.

Insertion of an Inflatable Implant

Implant surgeons have two approaches for inserting inflatable implants. The surgeon may choose the infrapubic approach or the penoscrotal approach. It's best if your surgeon is experienced in both techniques since sometimes during the implantation procedure, the surgeon must use an alternative surgical approach based on the patient's anatomy.

Dr. Paul Perito of Miami Beach, Florida, popularized the infrapubic approach to penile implantation. With this approach, the surgeon makes an incision above the penis, in the pubic area. The implant cylinders are inserted into the corporal cavernous bodies (shaft) of the penis; the reservoir is placed in the lower abdomen, and the pump is placed in the scrotum.

Dr. Steve Wilson of Fayetteville, Arkansas, popularized the penoscrotal approach, in which the implant device is inserted through a scrotal incision. As in the infrapubic approach, the reservoir is placed in the lower abdomen, the pump is placed in the scrotum, and the two cylinders are placed in the corporal cavernous bodies.

Insertion of a Semi-Rigid Implant

A subcoronal technique may be used for implanting a semi-rigid penile implant. With this method, the surgeon makes a small window just on the top of the penis, just behind the head, and the cylinders are inserted through this small window into the corporal cavernous bodies.

Taking Precautions

In all penile implant surgeries, we take many measures to minimize the chances of the implant becoming infected. Prior to the surgery, we recommend antibiotic preparation of the skin and intravenous antibiotic. During the procedure, we also wash the surgical operative site frequently with a specially prepared antibiotic solution.

Recovery from Surgery

Recovery time for the surgery is typically two to seven days; however, it will be four to six weeks before a man should engage in intercourse. Our recommendation is for early and frequent visits to your doctor during the postoperative period.

Postoperative Period

Postoperative discomfort is a normal side effect of the implant surgery. It is typically managed with pain medications. Other common side effects include bruising as well as swelling at the operative site. This is usually minimal in most patients and will resolve within several days after the procedure.

One of the potential complications of penile implant surgery is infection. We monitor a patient's incision closely to ensure that there is no development of a skin infection. Because of the care given before, during, and after the surgery, the penile implant has the lowest rate of infection, when compared to other human implants such as those used in breast and orthopedic surgeries.

We monitor the patient closely for swelling in the scrotum or bleeding within the scrotal sac, which is called a hematoma. We also make sure that the patient is urinating without difficulty.

Rarely, a revision surgery may be required. For example, if an implant should become infected or if an implant should start protruding through the skin or into the urethra, a revision surgery is needed to make a repair. These are extremely challenging procedures and should only be done by those surgeons who are highly trained in penile implant surgery.

Appearance with an Inflatable Implant

The appearance of a man's penis with a three-piece inflatable penile implant is natural, whether the penis is flaccid or erect. Each individual penile implant is "custom-fitted" to the patient's body during the surgical procedure. The implanting surgeon performs precise measurements and selects the appropriately sized implant for the patient. When the implant is deflated, the penis has a fuller, more-youthful appearance, and the penis does not retract.

Once an implant has been inserted, there is a possibility that you will have a decrease in the length of your penis in the flaccid state. The main reason for decreased length relates to the original condition that caused the erectile dysfunction. For example, if you have had ED for a long time, you may have lost some of the elasticity in the smooth muscle in the penis, causing a loss of length in the penis; if this is the case, you will not recover the length that you had as a young man.

Men need to remember that the implant cylinders sit in the corporal bodies of the penis and do not reach the glans, or the head of the penis. Accordingly, it is possible that when the implant is inflated and the penis becomes erect, the glans may swell in some men but not in all.

Sexual Function with an Inflatable Implant

We teach the patient and his partner how to use the inflatable implant device four to six weeks after the surgery. Management of expectations for a man receiving an implant is important. Education goes a long way toward making needed adjustments after a man has received a penile implant. Some men we have treated have been able to use the device sooner than the suggested four to six weeks; several men have needed to wait longer. The decision on how soon to use the implant is made by the physician.

Once a man is ready for sexual activity, he can achieve an erection by activating the pump in the scrotum, which transfers the fluid from the reservoir to the two cylinders in the corpora cavernosa. This causes the penis to become erect. This erection can be maintained as long as desired. When he's ready, the man can activate the pump release system, and the penis will return to its natural flaccid state.

Deflation of an Implant

Difficulty with inflation/deflation of the penile implant for patients is more often than not related to inadequate postoperative instructions. We spend more time giving the patients instructions when they experience this difficulty. We utilize an in-office model for practice that visually demonstrates how the device is inflated and deflated; we then have the man and then his partner demonstrate the inflation and deflation technique to us. Patients quickly become very comfortable with this technique.

The newest implant from Coloplast Corporation features two touch pads that offer one-touch release for deflation. When a man wants his penis to return the flaccid state, he simply uses his thumb and forefinger to depress the touch pads once and the implant deflates. Previous models required that a man hold the release bars until the implant fully deflated.

Auto-Inflation

It is rare that the penile implant will spontaneously inflate. This is called auto-inflation, and it is typically related to something that increases the pressure within the abdominal cavity, forcing fluid into the reservoir. Causes include such things as heavy lifting and straining, tight-fitting pants, constipation, or a full bladder. Auto-inflation may also occur in men who have had radical prostatectomy surgery or who have significant amounts of scarring in the penis from prior surgeries.

The implant device manufactured by Coloplast has developed a "lock-out valve," which significantly decreases the potential for auto-inflation. Surgeons can also help guard against auto-inflation by making sure that the space created for the reservoir is more than adequate, allowing the reservoir to expand to its full capacity.

Choosing an Implant Surgeon

The choice of the surgeon is probably one of the most important decisions that a patient will make with this type of surgery. Surgical experience is critical to the outcome. You should select a surgeon who performs more than ten procedures per year, has a low complication rate, and is willing to make a patient with an implant available to discuss his experience with you.

Does Insurance Pay for Implants?

Most, but not all, insurance companies cover the cost of penile implant surgery. Our advice is to check with your insurance company to determine if this surgery is covered prior to scheduling it. The support staff of the surgeon who will be performing the surgery should help with this.

There is currently a movement under way for passage of a federal law requiring all insurance companies to cover penile implant surgery for men who have undergone surgery or radiation treatment for prostate cancer. House Resolution 1903 would require that group and individual health insurance coverage and group health plans provide coverage for reconstructive prosthetic urology surgery if they provide coverage for prostate cancer treatment. The law would be similar to the one that federally mandated breast reconstruction for women who have had mastectomies.

Criticism of Penile Implants

Despite the improvements in penile implantation, there is a significant myth among a select group of physicians that the inflatable penile prostheses are fraught with surgical problems and are not a viable treatment alternative. In some cases, penile implants have been associated with surgical failure and/or patient complaints after surgery. Such concerns include:

- Infections
- Mechanical unreliability or failure
- Potential for decreased sensitivity after surgery
- Potential for loss of length of the penis after surgery
- Difficulty with inflation and/or deflation of the device
- Potential for spontaneous inflation
- Not always covered by insurance

However, the newest generation of implants has overcome these obstacles. Significant improvements have led to advanced training for implanting surgeons as well as advances in surgical techniques. Improvements have also been made with better patient selection, making sure a man is a good candidate for the procedure. Further, the implant devices have undergone a complete reengineering, and surgeons can apply antibiotic coatings to the devices, which reduces infection rates.

Simultaneous Surgery for Bladder Problems

Some men who are receiving implants may also wish to have their surgeons address other urological problems during their operation. For example, men who have had a radical prostatectomy may leak urine to some degree. This is often distressful to them. The newer procedures for the control of male urinary leakage include the insertion of artificial urinary sphincters and male slings; a sling keeps constant pressure on the urethra so that it does not open until the patient consciously releases the urine. Either of these procedures can be performed at the same time as the penile implant.

Also, treating Peyronie's disease with a penile implant is very popular. During this procedure, the implant device is inflated, and the curvature from the Peyronie's disease is straightened. Performing this procedure requires a high degree of surgical skill and should only be done by those surgeons who are highly trained in this procedure.

In Summary

If you are considering a penile implant, you should learn as much about the procedure as you can. Research the topic—read articles and search the Internet. Also, talk to patients who have implants. We find it very helpful to have our patients talk with our patient advocates, men who have undergone the penile implant procedure and are willing to talk frankly to others about their experience.

10

Safe Sex: It's Not Only
Avoiding STDs

B eing sexual is part of being a normal, healthy human. However, individuals with cardiovascular risks must take precautions to practice "safe sex." When we say safe sex, we're not talking about avoiding sexually transmitted diseases (STDs); we're referring to having sex without the risk of having a heart attack. This chapter is about cardiovascular risk factors and sexual activity. We want to clarify the guidelines for having sex safely, without the risk of a cardiovascular event.

Sex and Cardiac Risk Factors

The question of sexual activity and heart health is on the minds of many couples when a partner has cardiovascular risk factors. The research shows that energy exerted during sex with a familiar partner is not stressful on the heart. (The stress is no worse than in mild-to-moderate-intensity exercise for a middle-aged male.) The general rule that we follow in clinical practice is, "If you can walk up a flight of stairs without experiencing chest pain or severe shortness of breath, you can participate in sexual activity with your familiar partner in a familiar surrounding. Make that two flights of stairs if you're with an unfamiliar partner or in an unfamiliar setting."

However, the research on death during sexual activity has an interesting twist to it. Studies show that sex with an unfamiliar partner may increase the workload of the heart, especially if other factors are involved that are known to also increase this workload. These factors include such things as eating large meals and consuming alcohol.

To date, there have been three significant studies conducted on death during sex; these studies were done in Berlin, Frankfurt, and Japan. According to these studies, sudden, postcoital (after-sex) death had an incidence of less than 2 percent. Within this 2 percent of cases, extramarital sex accounted for more than 75 percent of the deaths. Men were the casualties more than 82 percent of the time.

Categories of Cardiac Risk

In 2004, the Princeton Consensus Conference on Sexual Dysfunction and Cardiac Risk gave health care providers clear and concise guidelines for evaluating the degree of cardiovascular risk associated with sexual activity for men who have varying degrees of cardiovascular disease.

According to the panel, major cardiovascular risk factors include: age, male gender, hypertension, diabetes mellitus, cigarette smoking, dyslipidemia, sedentary lifestyle, and a family history of premature coronary artery disease. Other risk factors include obesity, metabolic syndrome, elevated inflammatory markers, ethnicity, stress, and recreational drug use. The panel divided cardiovascular risk factors into three groups: low-risk patients, intermediate- or indeterminate-risk patients, and high-risk patients.

Low-Risk Patients

Low-risk cardiovascular patients can safely have sex. This group includes those with the following conditions:

- fewer than three of the major risk factors for cardiovascular disease and are asymptomatic (without any symptoms)
- hypertension or high blood pressure that is controlled with one or more medications
- well-controlled, mild, stable angina (chest pain)
- patients who have:
  - experienced a myocardial infarction (MI) more than six to eight weeks
  - revascularization (surgical repair) of the coronary arteries
  - mitral valve disease
  - left ventricular heart dysfunction or heart failure class I
  - other cardiovascular conditions such as controlled atrial fibrillation

Intermediate-Risk Patients

Intermediate- or indeterminate-risk patients were defined as those who have an uncertain cardiovascular condition. This group of people was advised to have further cardiac evaluation prior to resuming sexual activity. This group includes patients who:

- are asymptomatic (no symptoms) with more than three major risk factors
- have moderate stable angina
- had a heart attack less than six weeks ago and more than two weeks ago
- have left ventricular heart dysfunction class II
- have evident peripheral artery disease, stroke, and transient ischemic attacks

High-Risk Patients

The high-risk group of cardiac patients are people who are at significant risk for a cardiovascular event related to sexual activity. The symptoms in this category make individuals unstable, and they should not participate in sexual activity until their cardiac condition is stabilized. Diagnoses for this group include:

- unstable angina
- uncontrolled hypertension
- heart attack less than two weeks ago
- left ventricular dysfunction class III or IV and severe valvular disease, particularly aortic stenosis

If You Have High Blood Pressure

Having well-controlled hypertension, or high blood pressure, need not prevent a man from having sex. In fact, sexual activity is useful in controlling hypertension. However, uncontrolled hypertension is different, and sexual activity will place a person at risk for a cardiac event.

Some of the medications used to treat hypertension have the potential side effect of erectile dysfunction, but this cause of ED is easily treated. As mentioned earlier, the most common medications to treat hypertension, beta-blockers and thiazide diuretics, may in fact cause ED. The hypertension drugs least likely to cause ED are the newer angiotensin II receptor antagonists and alpha-blockers. (To review a list of the drugs in this categories, see chapter 5.)

If You Have Angina

Angina is pain in the chest caused by inadequate blood flow through the blood vessels of the heart. No matter the classification of the disorder, angina requires the heart to work harder. Even people with mild, stable angina requiring medical therapy should undergo further noninvasive evaluation prior to participating in sexual activity. Moderate stable angina increases the workload of the heart even more, and the risk of myocardial ischemia increases with sexual activity. Exercise testing is recommended prior to a cardiologist okaying sexual activity for people with moderate stable angina.

Any person experiencing unstable angina should be admitted to the hospital for evaluation and treatment. Anyone with this condition should not be sexually active until the angina is stabilized and he is cleared by a cardiologist for sexual activity.

Exterior of the Heart

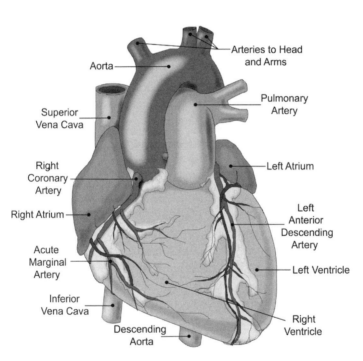

If You've Had a Heart Attack

Past myocardial infarction (MI), or heart attack, does not prevent a person from resuming sexual activity if he is at least six to eight weeks past the heart attack and is not having symptoms. Patients should seek clearance from a cardiologist to resume sexual relations any earlier than this, and getting such clearance would likely involve undergoing stress testing.

You can take precautions to prevent your heart from being overworked. For example, you can play a more-passive role during sexual activity and avoid activities that significantly increase the workload of the heart. Sexual activity should be resumed slowly. Foreplay, or pre-intercourse lovemaking, is essential, and we suggest that the patient start with gentle kisses, mutual petting, caresses, and cuddling. As you feel more confident, sexual activity can progress to penetration and intercourse. We do not recommend that the heart patient take an active, dominant role during intercourse. A comfortable side-by-side position is recommended. Slow down if any of these occur: chest pain, shortness of breath, increased heart rate, palpitations, anxiety, or other signs of distress.

If You've Had Heart Surgery

If you've had heart surgery to restore blood flow to the heart, it is recommended you have stress testing before resuming sexual activity. Restoring blood flow to the heart, called revascularization, is accomplished by different methods. The methods that the Princeton panel addressed were coronary artery bypass graft (CABG), and percutaneous coronary interventions such as stenting and angioplasty. A stent is a small metal device used to hold an artery open once it has been cleared. Angioplasty involves a surgical procedure in which a "balloon" is used to open clogged arteries.

On a related note, if you have had open-heart surgery, the sternal scar from surgery may be a source of pain, so we advise a side-by-side position or patient on top to minimize the discomfort. After a man has open-heart surgery, his chest hairs grow back bristly after surgery and may be uncomfortable for the partner. Positions in which the chest does not contact the partner's skin may be more comfortable; or placing fabric or a pillow between partners may be helpful.

If You Have Congestive Heart Failure

Left ventricular dysfunction and congestive heart failure need not prevent sexual activity if it is class I heart failure. Precautions must be taken if the disorder progresses into class II, III, or IV because these individuals are more at risk for developing an irregular heartbeat that could cause death. An implantable defibrillator or pacemaker decreases the risk for these life-threatening heartbeats. With the more-advanced classes of heart failure, symptoms may be the limiting factor for sexual activity. The partner with heart failure certainly should be the more-passive partner, frequently relying on the other partner to be more active during sex.

If You Have Heart Valve Disease

Valvular heart disease refers to disorders of the heart valves, which are the tissue flaps that regulate the flow of blood through the chambers of the heart. The mitral valve is located between the left atrium and the left ventricle. Mild mitral valvular disease is not a disorder that would prevent sexual activity.

The aortic valve is located between the left ventricle and the aorta. If a patient has significant aortic stenosis, or narrowing of the aortic valve, the risk of sudden death is higher and can be increased by the effects of vasodilators such as the PDE-5 inhibitors. Therefore, caution should also be used when taking PDE-5 inhibitors with aortic stenosis. Any man with valvular disease should consult his cardiologist about engaging in any sexual activity or strenuous activity.

If You've Had a Stroke

Cerebrovascular accidents, or strokes, occur more frequently at night or in early morning. Recent studies indicate that sexual activity not only does not increase the risk for stroke, but has actually demonstrated protection from cardiovascular events. If the couple was sexually active prior to the stroke, there are few reasons that would prevent the return of sex for the couple.

However, for the person who has experienced a stroke, resuming sexual activities can present many challenges because strokes are usually followed by decreased libido, depression, fatigue, and physical limitations. Starting off slowly with gentle kissing, touching, mutual petting, caressing, and cuddling is recommended. Urinary catheters can be removed from males and reinserted after sex, or folded back over the erect penis and covered with a prelubricated condom.

If total or partial paralysis is involved, the stroke victim should assume the more-passive role and the couple should select reasonable positions. Having the man who has suffered the stroke on his back with the partner on top is recommended; also recommended are side-by-side positions with added support for the stroke victim and the sitting position. We do not recommend the use of sex positions or sexual devices that require strength and coordination.

Are ED Drugs Safe for Cardiac Patients?

Questions about medication safety are frequently asked by people who have cardiovascular risk factors or a family history of cardiovascular disease. The question often on the minds of men with CVD and their partners is "How risky are the medications for the treatment of ED?"

There have been no studies that show the use of Viagra, Cialis, or Levitra are linked to heart attack or other cardiovascular events in men. Studies indicate that there are no changes in exercise EKG, workload of the heart, decrease in blood pressure, increase in cardiac ischemia, or increased heart rate with the use of these drugs.

Therefore, this classification of medications is not only safe, but may have benefits. Recent studies on Viagra have demonstrated cardiac benefits for endothelial function, improved cardiac output, and decreased blood pressure with patients who have pulmonary hypertension.

However, as we've stressed previously, these medications do have an interaction with nitrates and should not be taken with other medications containing nitrates. Men who develop chest pain after taking the PDE-5 inhibitors Viagra and Levitra are advised not to take nitroglycerin within twenty-four hours. Nitroglycerin should not be taken within forty-eight hours of taking Cialis. Men should not mix any of these ED drugs with amyl nitrate, a recreational inhalant called "poppers"; mixing this inhalant with ED drugs can cause a dangerous drop in blood pressure.

As we have stressed throughout this book, do not mix alpha-blockers and PDE-5 inhibitors. Talk to your doctor about this; we tell our patients not to take an alpha-blocker and a PDE-5 inhibitor within four hours of each other. As you may recall, alpha-blockers are a class of medication commonly used to treat an enlarged prostate, known as benign prostatic hyperplasia, or BPH. These medications also decrease blood pressure.

In Summary

We recommend and encourage a healthy sexual relationship for people with cardiovascular risk factors for both physical and psychological benefits. You would have to be very ill for the risk of sexual activity to outweigh the benefits. However, some people need to use caution and modify sexual techniques for physical safety reasons. And remember, the risk of having a heart attack increases if you don't know your partner. If you are an older male having sex with a partner outside of your familiar relationship, wearing a condom should not be your main concern.

11

Repair, Restore, and Rejuvenate Your Sex Life

Thomas A. Edison, U.S. inventor who lived from 1847 to 1931, once said, "The doctor of the future will give no medicine, but will interest her or his patients in the care of the human frame, in a proper diet, and in the cause and prevention of disease."

We are in agreement with Edison when we recommend lifestyle changes as part of the treatment for erectile dysfunction. There are several lifestyle factors that cause endothelial dysfunction, which in turn affects a man's erections. These factors include: smoking, increased cholesterol, hypertension, obesity, diabetes, and high-fat meals. As we've explained throughout this book, the relationship between cardiovascular disease and erectile dysfunction is well established and any lifestyle changes that a man makes to improve his cardiovascular health are going to improve the health of his penis.

Therapeutic Lifestyle Changes

In this chapter, we want to talk about rejuvenating your sex life, using therapeutic lifestyle changes (TLCs) for the treatment of erectile dysfunction. Making therapeutic lifestyle changes can restore and rejuvenate your sex life. These TLCs include:

- Exercise
- Lose weight
- Improve your diet
- Stop smoking
- Control blood glucose
- Control blood pressure
- Control lipid levels
- Communicate with your partner

Exercise

Exercise your way to a better sex life! Regular exercise improves libido, sexual confidence, and the ability to attain orgasm. Regular physical activity promotes psychological well-being and health.

Exercise extends the life span, helps with weight control, builds stronger bones, controls high blood pressure, lowers risk of cancer and depression, and improves mood. Reports from the American Heart Association, American College of Sports Medicine, Centers for Disease Control and Prevention, and the U.S. Surgeon General all stress that thirty minutes of low to moderate intensity exercise on most days of the week will reduce chronic diseases, decrease weight, and promote a healthy heart. To increase the return on exercise investment, increase the workout to forty-five to sixty minutes a day on most days of the week and limit caloric intake.

Exercise Helps Overcome ED

The New England Research Institutes studied 600 men over an eight-year period and reported on the effect of exercise on erectile dysfunction. This study concluded that there is a direct correlation between erectile dysfunction and physical activity: Men who had sedentary lifestyles had a higher risk of sexual dysfunction than those who exercised regularly. Taking a brisk two-mile walk or burning off 200 calories a day through exercise was most effective for reversing ED in some men.

There is also other research that makes the same point. In 1999, the American Medical Association reported that exercise increases the health of the cardiovascular system and can increase sexual potency. The report further states that good circulation is necessary for sexual function and that lifestyle behaviors such as smoking, heavy alcohol use, and obesity have a negative effect both on cardiovascular health and sexual potency. A recent study reaffirmed that physical activity provides an anti-inflammatory effect in the prevention of heart disease. The study concluded that there is an inverse relationship between physical activity and inflammatory markers such as C-reactive protein.

Numerous studies with obese men have concluded that a reduced-calorie diet combined with exercise can improve erectile dysfunction. In fact, physically active men over the age of fifty have reported better erections and have been found to have a 30 percent lower risk of ED than those who were physically inactive. Of all of the TLCs, exercising is the most important. Aim to exercise at least thirty minutes a day most days of the week.

Stronger Muscles Mean Better Sex

The benefits of cardiovascular exercise are well documented but other exercise that tones and builds muscle tissue will also have a positive effect on your sex life. Exercises that involve muscle groups of the pelvis, thighs, legs, and abdomen will increase sexual satisfaction. Even for men, Kegel exercises, in which you repeatedly tighten and squeeze the pelvic muscles, will strengthen and tone the muscles of the pelvic floor. These muscles support the urethra, bladder, penis, prostate, and rectum. It has been reported that the controlled contraction of the pelvic muscles improves the ability to achieve orgasm and is more pleasurable for the partner.

Therapeutic Lifestyle Recommendations

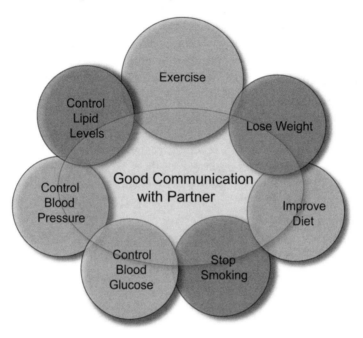

Squats, lunges, crunches, and leg lifts strengthen and tone the muscles necessary to develop muscular endurance and increase sexual stamina. There is an added benefit with weight training. Yoga increases flexibility that will enhance your sex life. These exercises will help you hold unusual positions longer.

Lose Weight

Losing weight is helpful in overcoming ED. A two-year Italian study done at an outpatient weight-loss clinic reported that a weight loss of 10 percent or more of body weight improved erectile function in obese men. This study looked at 110 obese men, ranging in age from thirty-five to fifty-five, with a body mass index (BMI) of 30 or greater; these men had significant ED. Body mass index refers to the number derived by using height and weight measurements to get a general indication if weight falls within a healthy range. (See BMI chart in the Appendix.)

The men in the study were randomly assigned to either a treatment group or a control group. The treatment group was given detailed counseling on increasing their physical activity and reducing total caloric intake. This group also met with an exercise trainer and nutritionist bimonthly for one year.

The control group received counseling on health, diet, and exercise at the beginning of the trial and at bimonthly visits to the clinic. However, they did not work with a trainer. At the end of the two-year study, the treatment group's average BMI had decreased from 36 to 31, a substantial improvement. Men in the treatment group also reported their erections had improved dramatically; their cardiac measurements improved as well.

Benefits of Weight Loss

- Ten percent weight loss improves erections in most men.
- For every thirty-five pounds a man loses he will gain approximately one inch of penile length.
- A four to ten pound weight loss lowers blood pressure 7/5 mm Hg.
- People with asthma who lost an average of thirty pounds over one year showed improved lung function.
- Losing as little as ten to fifteen pounds helps people with Type II Diabetes to better control their disease with less medication, and controlling weight can prevent getting Type II Diabetes.
- People with sleep apnea who lost as little as 10 percent of weight showed improved sleep patterns and had less daytime sleepiness.
- Decreasing weight by 5 to 10 percent can decrease risk for heart disease and stroke.

- Decreasing weight by 5 to 10 percent can decrease the risk for these cancers: In women: uterus, gallbladder, cervix, ovary, breast, and colon. In men: colon, rectum, and prostate.
- Weight loss of as little as ten pounds decreases the stress on hip, knee, ankle, and foot joints and lessens symptoms of osteoarthritis.
- Weight loss promotes improvement of lipids in the blood.

Improve Your Diet

A balanced, nutritious diet is crucial to good health. The diets that contribute most to clogging arteries are those that are high in saturated fats, carbohydrates, and trans-fatty acids; these foods leave deposits on the walls of the arteries, resulting in atherosclerosis. Unfortunately, this type of fatty diet is the one that most baby boomers grew up on. Multiple studies document that the traditional Western diet can be dramatically improved by following a diet similar to the Mediterranean diet.

The Mediterranean-style diet is associated with a lower risk of heart disease. Fewer people from the Mediterranean countries of Spain, Greece, and Italy die from cardiovascular disease compared to people in the United States or northern Europe.

Generally speaking, the Mediterranean diet is rich in fruits, vegetables, cereals, fish, and beans. It is also higher in total fat than other heart-healthy diets; however, the fats are

Best Foods for a Healthy Penis

- Apples
- Olive oil
- Peppers
- Celery
- Broccoli
- Salmon
- Garlic
- Soy
- Water
- Nuts
- Red wine

primarily monounsaturated (mostly olive oil) and omega-3 fats, those found in cold-water fish such as herring, salmon, tuna, and mackerel and in soybean and canola oils. Studies have shown that healthful fats may make platelets (clotting elements in the blood) less sticky and therefore less likely to clot. For diabetics, these fats can also help lower blood cholesterol better than the diets with higher carbohydrate counts.

The Mediterranean type of diet is good for both the heart and the penis. It emphasizes:

- Fresh fruits, vegetables, beans, nuts, seeds, and other plant foods
- Unrefined grains such as whole-grain cereals and breads
- Olive oil, rich in omega-9 fatty acids, as the major source of fat
- Alcohol in moderate amounts, mostly wine with meals
- Fresh wild-fish oil in moderate to high amounts
- Fresh fruits as the typical dessert, with honey or refined sugar several times a week
- Dairy products such as yogurt and cheese in low to moderate amounts
- Four or fewer eggs per week
- Reliance on fresh, locally produced foods and minimally processed foods
- Poultry in moderate to large amounts and red meat in low amounts
- Grilled, baked, or broiled foods instead of fried foods
- Unsalted nuts instead of salted nuts
- Water, water, water; fruit juices; sugar-free beverages instead of sweet beverages

Proteins

Choose lean proteins. Limit protein to no more than six ounces per day, and choose leaner cuts of meat, chicken, and fish instead of fatty meats. Beans and legumes are also good, low-fat sources of protein. Called the "wonder bean," soy products are some of the most nutritious foods on the planet. They are an excellent source of protein and fiber. Soy is found in tofu, miso, natto, tempeh, soy milk, soy flour, soybeans, soy nuts, and soy sauce. Soy can be purchased in liquid or powder form.

Carbohydrates

The best carbohydrates, complex carbohydrates, come from fresh, unprocessed fruits, vegetables, grains, and beans. These foods are important to a heart-healthy diet. They lower cholesterol levels and keep the blood flowing to the pelvic area. They are low in calories and aid in weight loss. Oat grains are the fiber of choice; research indicates that they can stimulate testosterone production.

Benefits of Omega-3

- Improves heart health, reduces arrhythmia, reduces triglycerides
- Lowers high blood pressure
- Improves brain health
- Improves rheumatoid arthritis
- Helps prevent cancer
- Controls GI–ulcerative colitis
- Helps control insulin levels in Type II Diabetes
- Helps control asthma and COPD (chronic obstructive pulmonary disease)
- Decreases pain and inflammation
- Helps prevent skin problems such as psoriasis

"Bad" Fats

There is often confusion about which fats are good for us and which ones are bad. First, let's note that all fats are relatively high in calories. However, some fats are good for our bodies; other fats are not.

The so-called bad fats are saturated fats that come from animal products, such as meat and dairy products, and from tropical oils, such as palm and coconut oils. The American Heart Association recommends that you get no more than 7 percent of your daily fat calories from saturated fats. These fats can clog arteries and slow or even prevent the flow of blood to the heart and to the genital tissue.

Other bad fats, trans fats, are found in hydrogenated and partially hydrogenated oils used in food processing. These oils are often used in processed foods to extend their shelf life; they are found in such foods as potato chips, commercial salad dressing, margarine, crackers, cookies, and many packaged baked goods

"Good" Fats

Monounsaturated fats are the good fats; they are the best source of fat for your heart and the production of hormones. Monounsaturated fats are primarily found in such foods as olive oil, canola oil, peanut oil, sunflower oil, sesame oil, avocados, and many seeds and nuts. These fats do not appear to affect cholesterol and, in fact, may help lower blood cholesterol levels.

Another good fat, polyunsaturated fat, is usually of plant origin. Foods high in polyunsaturated fat include a number of vegetable oils, including soybean oil, corn oil, and safflower oil, as well as fatty fish such as salmon, mackerel, herring, and trout. These fish contain the highly beneficial omega-3 fats.

Other sources of polyunsaturated fat include some nuts and seeds. Despite their high fat content, studies have shown that eating walnuts every day can lead to a 12 percent drop in total cholesterol and a 16 percent drop in LDL, the bad cholesterol. Walnuts are also high in omega-3 fatty acids and keep the vascular system healthy. They also contain other nutrients good for the heart, such as zinc, folic acid, vitamin E, and magnesium.

Read Food Labels

Food labels are important in the quest for healthy eating, but they can be confusing to read for the novice. Food labels are all set up the same way; they do not vary by product or manufacturer. There are six extremely important areas of information that you must know when selecting heart- and sex-healthy food:

- Calories per serving, or total calories, should be enough to maintain ideal body weight. There are nine calories per gram of fat, four calories per gram of carbohydrate, and four calories per gram of protein.
- Total fat should be less than 30 percent of your total daily calories.
- Saturated fat should be less than 7 percent of total calories; it will raise your blood cholesterol and increase your risk for heart disease.
- Trans fats are now listed on all food labels.
- Cholesterol should be kept to less than 300 mg per day.
- About five to ten grams of soluble fiber or roughage should be consumed per day.

Supplements for Sexual Health

Pycnogenol alone or combined with L-arginine are antioxidants that have been recommended as nutritional supplements that will enhance heart health as well as sexual health. They shield the endothelium lining of the blood vessels of the body and enable better nitric oxide utilization.

Pycnogenol works by neutralizing free radicals which oxidize LDL cholesterol, keeping blood platelets from becoming too sticky and forming clots at plaque sites, protecting endothelium, and decreasing blood pressure by inhibiting the constriction of blood vessels.

L-arginine works by helping the body to build protein and is the only amino acid that is a nitric oxide generator. You'll recall, nitric oxide in the blood is required for achieving an erection. Nitric oxide builds muscles, aids in the release of growth hormone, aids in the fight against cancers, and helps battle infections.

Stop Smoking

If you don't smoke, don't start. If you do smoke, quit. As emphasized earlier, smoking has been well documented as a major risk factor for the development of cardiovascular disease and erectile dysfunction. It can also cause infertility. Although we don't have a great deal of scientific data on how smoking cessation relates to a man's recovery from ED, we have seen men in our practice who have had some recovery of erectile function when they stopped smoking. There are clinical studies that demonstrate the complete reversal of nicotine damage to the penis.

According to the American Cancer Society, as soon as you snuff out that last cigarette, your body begins a series of physiological changes.

Benefits of Smoking Cessation

- Within twenty minutes: Blood pressure, body temperature, and pulse rate will drop to normal.
- Within eight hours: Smoker's breath disappears. Carbon monoxide level in blood drops, and oxygen level rises to normal.
- Within twenty-four hours: Chance of heart attack decreases.
- Within forty-eight hours: Nerve endings start to regroup. Ability to taste and smell improves.
- Within three days: Breathing is easier.

- Within two to three months: Circulation improves. Walking becomes easier. Lung capacity increases up to 30 percent.
- Within one to nine months: Sinus congestion and shortness of breath decrease. Cilia that sweep debris from your lungs grow back. Energy increases.
- Within one year: Excess risk of coronary heart disease is half that of a person who smokes.
- Within two years: Heart attack risk drops to near normal.
- Within five years: Lung cancer death rate for the average former pack-a-day smoker decreases by almost half. Stroke risk is reduced. Risk of mouth, throat, and esophageal cancer is half of that of a smoker.
- Within ten years: Lung cancer death rate is similar to that of a person who does not smoke. The precancerous cells are replaced.
- Within fifteen years: Risk of coronary heart disease is the same as for a person who never smoked.

Source: American Cancer Society, *Guide for Quitting Smoking*

Health professionals need to work with smokers to help them find a way to kick the habit. Many people find it helpful to use the nicotine replacement products now available in several forms. These include chewing gum, inhalers, nasal spray, and patches, which are applied to the skin.

Medication for Smoking Cessation

The drug buproprion, sold as *Zyban*, can help with smoking cessation. The drug lessens the unpleasant withdrawal symptoms that a smoker experiences when nicotine is no longer entering the bloodstream. A newer drug, varenicline, marketed as *Chantix*, is a non-nicotine medication that shows promise for those wishing to stop smoking. In a twelve week test, 44 percent of the participants were able to kick the habit.

For a Better Sexual Life: Suggestions that Work!

1. Connect before you caress, do things alone together that make you feel closer. At least weekly, spend an uninterrupted hour doing something that is fun or mutually satisfying (take a walk, have brunch, see a romantic movie).

2. Don't forget romancing outside the bedroom—court each other.

3. Plan time together (when children arrive, or life intrudes, spontaneity leaves). Make a "date to make love."

4. Create privacy. Lock the door, turn off the TV and (cell) phones.

5. Sex is adult play. Be sensual—let your skin and senses wake up to touch and caress. Use oils or powder so that your hands glide.

6. Don't expect mind reading—let your partner know what you like—the kind of touch, the movements, the pace you enjoy.

7. Stay positive and constructive—criticism never made anyone a better lover.

8. Think about enhancing the variety of your sexual activities. Occasionally try something "new" or slightly "forbidden." Pretend you've just met, take a shower or bath together, put on something sexy.

9. Forgive easily. Don't let the little things ruin sexual intimacy.

10. Keep your sense of humor—things often go wrong. Humor is the best lubricant.

11. Make your partner feel valued. Give a gift of yourself every day. A word of praise or compliment, hug or caress outside the bedroom, a flower, a card, special food, a few minutes of your full attention, your special helpfulness. A loving connection is the most important goal.

Reprinted with permission by Drs. Marian Dunn and Sandra Leiblum.

Control Blood Sugar

Several studies show that optimal blood glucose management not only leads to a healthier heart but to a healthier penis and a healthier erection as well. Management of blood glucose through diet and exercise is ideal. However, if you are diabetic, you'll require additional medical therapy to achieve control.

Control Blood Pressure

Once again, management of hypertension through diet and exercise is ideal. Diet changes should include sodium restrictions. Sodium or salt intake should be kept to 2,300 milligrams per day or less if you have high blood pressure. Some blood pressure medications can adversely affect your sexual function. Please consult with your health care provider prior to starting or stopping any medication.

Control Lipid Levels

Studies have indicated that optimizing lipid levels can have a positive effect on prevention of erectile dysfunction and optimizing sexual function. Please consult with your health care provider and be aware of your lipid levels.

Communicate with Your Partner

Sexual dysfunction is not just an individual's problem. It is a couple's problem. It is important for each partner to remember that sex is important to both of them and that communicating about ED or other sexual problems is essential to overcoming the problem. Ignoring the problem will not lead to resolution. Here are some tips for communicating with your partner about sexual dysfunction.

DO:	DON'T:
• communicate with understanding and compassion.	• be critical or place blame on one partner or the other.
• give reassurance and express love for each other often.	• focus on the sexual dysfunction disorder in daily interactions with your partner.
• be supportive.	• criticize, judge, get defensive, or take or give blame.
• continue loving your partner.	• stop being affectionate, accept excuses, or feel as if the love is gone from the relationship.
• be active in the treatment process.	• ignore or avoid the problem.

Express yourself to your partner in a supportive and loving manner. You might say, "Sex is important to me, and I'd like for us to handle the problem together as a couple." It's important to select the best environment for talking about intimacy issues. Select a time when you will be uninterrupted and when there will be enough time to fully discuss the issues. Use the time to share honestly and openly so that the time together will make you feel emotionally closer to each other.

Remember that sexual dysfunction is a medical condition that can be treated. There is a range of treatments available, from pills to surgical procedures, and doctors will work with couples to find the best successful treatment option for them.

Seek Therapy If Needed

The success of communication between couples is influenced by many factors. These factors include basic assumptions about the disorder and treatments, current beliefs or standards of the couple, expectations of treatment outcomes, and feelings of confidence or resentment. When barriers to communication are apparent, we often recommend therapy with a multidisciplinary team that might include any of several disciplines: urology, primary care, pharmacology, endocrinology, cardiology, neurology, psychiatry, counseling, and perhaps sex therapy.

Members of such teams have expertise to help couples identify core problems and to facilitate the couple's developing methods of coping and overcoming the problems. It is through this team approach that many of the couples we have treated have found their way back to enjoying a life filled with intimacy and sexual fulfillment.

What About Aphrodisiacs?

In 1989, the Food and Drug Administration proclaimed that there is scientific proof that over-the-counter, self-proclaimed aphrodisiacs may actually improve sexual function, despite the lack of controlled studies. Horny goat weed, which has been used in China for more than 2,000 years, has been reported to increase libido. Other well-known aphrodisiacs include oysters, alcohol, chocolate, ginger, spices, and yohimbine.

Oysters

Oysters are high on the list of aphrodisiacs. One of history's most famous lovers, Casanova, was reported to eat fifty oysters a night at dinner. Zinc, found abundantly in oysters, is an essential nutrient for a healthy sex life. A large amount of zinc is found in the male ejaculate. Zinc deficiencies can contribute to decreased sperm count, lowered testosterone levels, and prostate problems. Other foods high in zinc include beans, cashews, raisins, dates, fish, chicken, lamb, pork, and veal.

Alcohol in Moderation

If used in moderation, alcohol can promote a healthy heart, ease inhibition, and provoke desire. The *Dietary Guidelines for Americans* define moderate drinking as no more than one alcoholic drink a day for women and no more than two alcoholic drinks a day for men. One drink equals 5 ounces of wine, 12 ounces of beer, 1.5 ounces of 80 proof distilled spirits, or 1 ounce of 100 proof distilled spirits. Red wine contains resveratrol and other antioxidants that have been proven to reduce heart disease. Research is ongoing to determine the benefits of wine for increasing HDL (the good cholesterol) and its antioxidant and anticoagulant qualities.

However, alcohol in excess can be the cause of erectile dysfunction, increased triglycerides, high blood pressure, and heart failure. Long-term alcohol abuse can cause permanent, irreversible erectile dysfunction in men.

Chocolate in Moderation

Chocolate is truly a gift from the gods. It can be sensual and have real, positive benefits to your sex life. It contains phenylethylamine, a chemical that releases dopamine in the brain, producing a feeling of well-being or euphoria. Dark chocolate, when taken in moderation and in the form of pure cocoa, has antioxidant properties and can be beneficial for your heart. What could be better than chocolate cookies with walnuts? Of course, moderation is key. Overindulgence leads to obesity and may contribute to brittle bones.

Ginger

Ginger has been used in many cultures for a number of remedies for more than 600 years. It has been reported to help with gastric upset, headaches, and other medical problems. Research indicates that ginger keeps the blood from clotting, much the same as aspirin. Ginger acts as a stimulant for the circulatory system, thus increasing blood flow to the genitals. The plant may be made into a tea, added to recipes, or ingested as a powder.

Spicy Foods

Spicy foods containing capsaicin are reported to stimulate the release of endorphins. Endorphins, a morphine-like substance within the brain, were discovered in 1975. They reduce stress and pain, enhance the immune system, and delay the aging process. Endorphin release is responsible for the "runner's high," the feeling of euphoria associated with continuous exercise such as running, skiing, aerobics, or cycling.

Sex and endorphins are linked as well. Recent studies indicate that the production of endorphins increases as much as 200 percent with sexual activity. Clinical studies from Johns Hopkins University concluded that there is a positive correlation between endorphin release and orgasm.

Hot peppers also contain vitamin C and chemicals called flavonoids, which protect your heart. One flavonoid found in hot peppers is quercetin, which lowers LDL, the bad cholesterol. Quercetin is helpful in relieving pelvic pain, as well. Habanera peppers are the hottest of the chilies, thereby producing the most endorphins. Other hot peppers containing high levels of capsaicin include jalapeño and cayenne.

Yohimbine

Yohimbine is from the bark of a South American tree. It may possess properties that act on the nervous system, in particular the nerves in the spine that control erections.

There is clinical evidence of yohimbine's aphrodisiac effect. It is a weak alpha-adrenergic blocker. Men who took it reported improvement with psychological erectile dysfunction. Yohimbine can be found in most health food stores. However, using the herb can be extremely dangerous if you have heart disease, take it in large doses, or mix it with other medications.

In Summary

Finally, we stress again that what is good for the heart is good for the penis. As Dr. Steven Lamm, author of *The Hardness Factor*, states, "the harder the erection, the healthier the man."

Restore, repair, and rejuvenate your sex life with the TLCs listed in this chapter. Always consult your clinician prior to starting or stopping a medication or vitamin supplement.

PART IV

Women and Sexual Dysfunction

12

Female Sexual Dysfunction

As a woman, do you have a sexually satisfying life with your partner? Chances are you're answering "no," since an estimated 30 to 50 percent of females suffer from some version of female sexual dysfunction. Unfortunately, most women do not seek treatment for sexual dysfunction unless the problem is causing personal distress.

Female sexual dysfunction is a broad term for several disorders involving arousal, orgasm, sexual desire, and/or pain that result in extreme personal distress. The problem may have been present throughout a woman's life, or she may have acquired the problem later on. Read on to learn more about this spectrum of problems.

It's a Woman's Problem, Too

Sexual dysfunction is as much a health issue for women as erectile dysfunction is for men. You may not realize it since much of the media hype in this area focuses almost solely on medications to help men with their performance issues. But with 50 percent of women complaining that they've experienced at least one manifestation of sexual dysfunction, it's clear that they, too, could benefit from medical help. What's more, if there is a problem, it's likely to get worse with age.

Although many women cite the lack of a partner as the number one reason for not engaging in satisfying sexual activity when they're older, there are many other factors that come into play. Ranging from a partner's age and sexual function to the atrophy of sexual organs and decreased muscle tone, the list includes hypertension, diabetes mellitus, arthritis, stroke, chronic pain, and even lack of privacy. All of these issues can diminish desire and function. The situation is complicated by the fact that sexual function and sexual desire in women are strongly intertwined. It's often difficult to determine which issue came first.

These and other underlying disorders may or may not have a negative effect on someone's health or quality of sexual life. But when they do cause personal distress, it's time for a woman to seek treatment. Since female sexual dysfunction, like erectile dysfunction, has ties to cardiovascular disease, getting help does more than just improve your sexual activity. It just may save your life.

Sexual Satisfaction Is Key for Both Genders

The concept that sexuality is an important part of a woman's life has not changed since Alfred Kinsey first suggested the idea in 1948. His pioneering research concerning all aspects of human sexuality gave both men and women, particularly women in menopause, a better understanding of their intimate lives.

From his work, and that of other scientists, we know that sexuality and sexual activity (from cuddling to intercourse) are important to both men and women even as they age. One study suggests that 47 percent of women, ages sixty-six to seventy-one, remain sexually active, while 28 percent of those older than seventy-eight want to stay in the game.

Still, a lack of reliable testing tools and evidence-based studies makes diagnosing female sexual dysfunction challenging for both physician and patient. Doctors must rely on laboratory screens for other potential underlying health issues rather than a specific test confirming female sexual disorder. What's more, there are few valid studies concerning the treatment of female sexual dysfunction. This is further complicated by the lack of distinction between what's normal and abnormal.

Continued research is needed to develop better diagnostic tools and treatment guidelines. Until then, an increasing number of female baby boomers will have to rely on what we do know to help them achieve more-satisfying sexual lives.

Categories of Female Sexual Dysfunction

Although sexual problems are widespread in both genders, female sexual dysfunction has been identified as a health problem only recently. In its *Diagnostic and Statistical Manual of Mental Disorders*, Fourth Edition (*DSM-IV*), the American Psychiatric Association divides female sexual dysfunction into the four categories that follow.

Low Libido Disorder

Affecting approximately 40 percent of females, hypoactive or low sexual desire is the leading sexual dysfunction complaint among women. It's characterized by a diminished or complete lack of: libido, interest in initiating sex, or fantasizing about sex. Women affected with this problem don't desire sexual stimulation or respond to it. In rare instances, they may also suffer from sexual aversion, a pronounced distaste for or avoidance of sexual contact. This condition is often triggered by sexual or physical trauma and abuse.

Low libido, on the other hand, may be a common side effect of selective serotonin reuptake inhibitors and other medications used to treat depression. It also becomes progressively common with aging, even though the problems we're discussing here go beyond what's normal. Diminished

Carol's Story

Carol, an outgoing fifty-seven-year-old, accompanied her husband Bob to our office; he was being treated for erectile dysfunction. As we worked through the process, Carol suddenly admitted one day that she didn't mind the lack of sexual intimacy with her husband because she experienced pain during intercourse. She thought it was a natural part of aging, so she was hesitant about Bob's treatment. If it worked, their sexual activity would resume, and that just meant more discomfort.

Once Carol shared her fears, however, we could address her role in this couple's issues with intimacy. Our examination revealed that Carol had low estrogen levels with vaginal atrophy and dryness. With topical estrogen replacement and a vaginal dilator, however, she could experience intimacy without feeling pain. With the help of her secretions and, occasionally, a water-soluble lubricant, having sex was no longer an unwanted event. Once Bob overcame his erectile dysfunction with appropriate treatment, the two could enjoy sexual intimacy again.

sexual desire occurs in an estimated 10 percent of women age forty-nine or younger; in an estimated 22 percent, ages fifty to sixty-five; and in an estimated 47 percent, ages sixty-six to seventy-four.

Female Sexual Arousal Disorder

Similar to erectile dysfunction in men, sexual arousal disorder in women is the inability to achieve and progress through the normal stages of arousal. This category is divided into three areas: Genital sexual arousal disorder occurs when your vulva doesn't engorge during intimacy and your vagina isn't lubricated enough for penile penetration. One cause is believed to be reduced blood flow to the area. Subjective sexual arousal disorder is the absence or decrease in sexual excitement, arousal, or pleasure from any form of stimulation. Combined genital and subjective arousal disorder is a blend of both conditions.

Female Orgasmic Disorder

A common sexual dysfunction in women, anorgasmia is characterized by a markedly diminished intensity during orgasm after "normal" arousal. It may also mean a woman has a delayed or absent orgasm. Often linked to common antidepressants, female orgasmic disorder doesn't appear to be age related and is not a part of the normal aging process. Research suggests that 25 percent of women in the United States ages eighteen to seventy-four experience some form of orgasmic dysfunction. Uncontrolled or poorly controlled hypertension is an additional risk factor with orgasmic disorders.

Dyspareunia

Defined as genital pain, before, during, or after intercourse, dyspareunia is characterized by persistent or recurrent discomfort with every attempted or actual penetration of the vagina by a penis. The pain may be deep or superficial. One of the least-common dysfunctions, this sexual pain is typically related to other conditions such as surgical or obstetric injury and vaginal atrophy. Although it can be superficial, it often manifests itself as a deep pain caused by the penis nudging or putting pressure on an ovary and/or the cervix. But your doctor will have many potential sources to rule out since dyspareunia can be caused by a host of health problems, from physical and sexual abuse to genital herpes and other sexually transmitted diseases.

The remaining list of possible causes includes such things as hormone deficiencies, mechanical or chemical irritation, hemorrhoids, urethritis, radiation therapy, irritable bowel syndrome, urinary tract infections, spermicides, or the size of your partner's penis. Whatever the source of dyspareunia, identifying it is essential for successful treatment.

Female Sexual Dysfunction–Cardiac Link

Just as it is in men, sexual dysfunction in women may be an early sign of cardiovascular disease. Research has shown that the link between cardiac disease and female sexual dysfunction is similar to that of heart disease and male erectile dysfunction. In fact, by understanding the physiology and treatment success of ED, clinicians have a better grasp of female sexual dysfunction.

Doctors know, for instance, that when the heart can't pump blood efficiently to the body's organs, those organs, including the genitals, can't function optimally. In terms of sexual function, less efficiency can lead to decreased desire, decreased arousal, and decreased ability to achieve orgasm. It can also result in painful intercourse due to lack of lubrication.

What has research shown us about coronary artery disease and female sexual dysfunction? A number of things. Women with coronary artery disease are more likely than healthy women to suffer female sexual dysfunction. One study demonstrated that 60 percent of participants with coronary problems had some form of female sexual dysfunction, as compared to 33 percent of the healthy women followed. Coronary patients displayed a significant decrease in sexual function in all applicable areas, including arousal, lubrication, and orgasm.

Blood Flow to Genitals Is Diminished

Vascular insufficiency decreases the blood flow to the clitoral and vaginal areas, leading to diminished lubrication and arousal as well as painful intercourse. A decrease in pelvic blood flow, caused by diseases of the aorta or iliac vessels (or trauma to pelvic floor structures), also can foster the formation of excess connective tissue (called smooth muscle fibrosis), which leads to vaginal dryness and painful sex.

Cardiovascular Medications and Impaired Sexual Function

Uncontrolled hypertension and antihypertensive medications are associated with decreased lubrication of the vagina, dyspareunia, and orgasmic disorders. Among women who experienced a myocardial infarction, approximately 44 percent reported a decline in the frequency of sexual intercourse; 27 percent reported total abstinence. Sexual arousal disorder is the most common sexual problem in women after coronary artery bypass surgery.

Metabolic Syndrome Is a Factor

Women who exhibit metabolic syndrome, a collection of risk factors for heart disease, also are at higher risk for female sexual dysfunction. In a recent study of 200 premenopausal women, ages twenty to forty-eight, 120 participants with metabolic syndrome reported significantly more difficulty with sexual arousal, orgasm, and lubrication than the 80 without the syndrome. Women with the syndrome reported an overall decrease in sexual satisfaction.

Diagnosis May Be Complicated

Diagnosing female sexual dysfunction requires a comprehensive approach, including both physical and laboratory examinations plus a complete medical and psychosexual history. Since we believe every sexual issue is a couple's issue, treatment is more successful if your partner actively participates in the process. Involving your spouse or significant other not only facilitates the diagnosis but also helps in fixing the problem. History has shown us that treatment plans for sexual dysfunction are more successful if both partners are committed to finding a solution.

So what can you expect from the diagnostic process? Your clinician will investigate a variety of topics after first doing a medical history. His or her goal is to formulate a complete picture of the factors that might be causing your sexual distress. You'll be discussing current and past health issues, including any history of trauma or psychiatric problems, along with any medications you might be taking. Your doctor will also address the nature and duration of your symptoms as well as the level of distress they're causing.

Evaluation for Sexual Dysfunction

In addition to examining your genital area, it is very important that the doctor screen you for other conditions that can cause sexual dysfunction. From neurological disorders and depression to metabolic syndrome and cardiovascular disease, the list of potential issues linked to female sexual dysfunction is extensive. It may include genitourinary disorders, diabetes mellitus and other endocrine dysfunctions, menopause, and chronic pain. The dysfunction may also be a side effect of medications for health problems such as hypertension.

To identify the most successful treatment plan, your doctor will want to screen carefully for these underlying problems. He or she will also order follow-up tests according to your symptoms. Among the baseline screens you can expect are a complete blood count, a comprehensive metabolic profile, a fasting glucose and cholesterol analysis, and hormone tests for testosterone, thyroid, estrogen, prolactin, and DHEA levels.

Checking for Bladder Problems

Your physician will want to make sure that any urinary tract symptoms you may be experiencing are also addressed. Problems such as overactive bladder, interstitial cystitis, and stress urinary incontinence may need to be treated and controlled for you to enjoy sexual intimacy.

An overactive bladder, in particular, can cause a significant decrease in quality of life for women. But although it can be a troubling root of female sexual dysfunction, it can also be treated with various anticholinergic/antimuscarinic medications, drugs that block the nerves involving the bladder and control its muscle contractions. Many of the newer agents don't have the same drying effect of older drugs and therefore don't result in decreased lubrication.

Your doctor will also want to treat any signs of interstitial cystitis. More than one-fifth of all women diagnosed with this chronic inflammation of the bladder wall also report painful intercourse. More than one-third of them completely abstain from sex because of the discomfort. So controlling the symptoms can be very helpful to your sexual health.

In addition, new medications and surgical interventions can easily correct stress urinary incontinence, a condition that impacts your physiological well-being, including the ability to have sex. A recent study demonstrated that about 40 percent of women have sexual dysfunction associated with their urinary tract issues.

Male Performance Factor

How satisfied is the woman with the performance of her male partner? The man's performance needs to be considered. We know, for instance, that when a man enjoys a healthy sex life (and is able to achieve an erect penis), both he and his partner will have an enhanced experience. A 2005 study of 229 couples in which the men were being treated for erectile dysfunction showed that addressing the erection issues in these men improved the sexual satisfaction and function in their female partners even though these partners had no changes in arousal, desire, or orgasm. We've seen similar grateful patients and their partners in our own practice. When we have successfully treated a man's erectile dysfunction, his partner typically expresses gratitude at having regained an active sexual relationship.

Treatment for Women

Treating female sexual dysfunction works best when we approach the problem as a partner issue. As with erectile dysfunction in men, we find our best outcomes occur when both people are actively engaged in the diagnosis and treatment plan. That means making sure that our patients and their partners understand the causes of female sexual dysfunction, the correct steps to diagnose it, and the best treatment plans.

Since educating patients is central to achieving positive results, we encourage every couple to read and investigate this condition on their own. The treatment of female sexual dysfunction is evolving as scientists target their research sights on the topic and develop even more evidence-based guidelines. Besides helping a woman maintain a healthy heart, we can offer other forms of treatment for sexual dysfunction.

Estrogen Replacement

If your female sexual dysfunction is related to menopause, your physician may suggest estrogen replacement. Not only can it relieve the hot flashes associated with your body's midlife changes, but it also will improve genital sensation and decrease both burning and pain with sexual intercourse. Estrogen can be taken as an oral medication or via a topical cream, patch, or ring inserted into the vagina. The lowest dosage necessary to achieve symptom relief is recommended.

Testosterone Replacement

Testosterone replacement is an effective yet challenging way to lessen some of the symptoms associated with female sexual dysfunction. Just as low testosterone levels in men can contribute to erectile dysfunction, low levels of testosterone in women can also affect sexual function and sex drive. The upside is that replacing this hormone can yield a variety of positive results, including increased libido, energy, and feelings of well-being. It can also improve vaginal lubrication while relaxing vaginal tissue. The downside is that laboratory testing methods to evaluate testosterone levels in women are based on the much higher concentrations found in men. Moreover, guidelines to determine "normalcy" in pre- and postmenopausal women are determined by test values of women without female sexual dysfunction.

In addition to difficulties associated with laboratory analysis, there are also side effects with replacement testosterone. Many women experience menstrual irregularities, an enlarged clitoris, and increased hair growth, along with acne and oily skin. Although these side effects occur mostly with high doses, they can surface with lower amounts as well. Many women find all the above unacceptable and may discontinue use. If you're interested in testosterone replacement, however, you'll find it's available for "off-label" use in the form of tropical gels and creams to oral medications.

Eros-Clitoral Therapy Device

The first treatment approved by the Food and Drug Administration for arousal and orgasmic disorders in women, the Eros-Clitoral Therapy Device is a small handheld device that fits onto the clitoris. It's designed to increase blood flow to the clitoris and surrounding tissue by vacuuming the tissue gently. Clinical studies report arousal and orgasmic improvements in pre- and postmenopausal women using the device. Designed to fit on the fingertip and be used with a lubricant, the Vielle Clitoral Stimulator makes orgasms easier to obtain and more satisfying by increasing blood flow to the clitoris and surrounding area.

Viagra

Approved by the FDA to treat both erectile dysfunction and pulmonary arterial hypertension, Viagra is not approved for female sexual dysfunction. However, some animal studies have shown that the drug relaxes the clitoral and vaginal smooth muscles. Other research has demonstrated benefits with antidepressant-induced sexual dysfunction in women. More studies are needed to gauge the effectiveness of this drug in women. Meanwhile, use of these types of drugs are "off label."

Zestra

Herbal products such as *Zestra,* a natural botanical oil, reportedly enhance sexual function in women. When gently massaged onto the female genitalia three to five minutes prior to sexual intercourse, it can increase levels of desire, arousal, satisfaction, and sexual pleasure.

In Summary

The number of untreated women with female sexual dysfunction remains high and will no doubt climb with the aging of the baby boom generation. As science reveals more information about this condition, however, we hope their efforts lead to better and better treatment plans. In time, clinical trials are likely to yield new information about effective agents, giving us many more options to offer women suffering from sexual dysfunction.

In Closing

We hope this book has given you some insights about the important relationship between the health of your heart and the health of your sex life. As we have said all through this book, sexual dysfunction, especially ED, can be a harbinger of cardiovascular disease. By aggressively managing cardiovascular risk factors, you are aggressively managing your risk factors for erectile dysfunction.

The last decade has ushered in exciting new treatment forms, namely the PDE-5 inhibitors. Given the properties of these drugs, it is conceivable that many of us will be taking one of these PDE-5 inhibitors in the next decade for prevention and protection from the ravages of aging, pulmonary hypertension, prostate hyperplasia, stroke, Peyronie's disease, or priapism.

And the future holds even more possibilities. We will likely see the development of more types of PDE-5 inhibitors that are faster-acting and have more-optimal duration, as well as receptor selectivity to increase potency. Medications to stimulate the brain to achieve erections are already in clinical testing. Other advances will be topical medications that are rubbed on the penis. The testing for endothelial function or dysfunction and the correlation to erectile dysfunction for the individual will be more readily available and have a role in ED management. The surgical arena for treatment of erectile dysfunction has stabilized. The penile implant is probably the best surgical option available. The placement of these implants has never been safer or more effective. The devices have had multiple modifications to prevent the most-dreaded complication, infection, and the incidence of infection is at an all-time low. The design and function of the implant has stayed essentially the same over time; the penile implant is the least-revised implant placed in the human body, much less so than those for hips, knees, and valves.

The reengineering of the penile implant release valves has been accomplished and allows for deflation with minimal effort.

Finally, we predict that there will be a whole host of research and treatments for female sexual dysfunction, including topical medications to improve local blood flow. Remember, the risk factors for sexual dysfunction in men also apply to women.

Appendix A

Medications that can cause Sexual Dysfunction

Antihypertensive: Associated with decreased libido, decreased arousal and orgasmic disorder in women. Associated with decreased libido, decreased arousal, orgasmic disorder and erectile dysfunction in men. Commonly used medications are:

Beta Blockers:

- Inderal
- Tenormin
- Blocadren
- Corgard
- Lopressor
- Toprol

Calcium Channel Blockers:

- Adalat
- Cardizem XR
- Isoptin
- Verelan
- Calan
- Tiazac
- Procardia
- Dilacor

Alpha Blockers:

- Doxazosin
- Prazosin
- Terazosin

Diuretics:

- Diuril
- Aldactone
- Lasix

Medications used to treat depression, anxiety and sedatives: Associated with erectile dysfunction, orgasmic disorders in men and orgasmic disorders, loss of sexual desire and arousal in women. Commonly used medications are:

145

Antidepressants:

- Prozac
- Luvox
- Norpramin
- Mellaril
- Anafranil
- Sinequan

- Zoloft
- Serzone
- Prolixin
- Nardil
- Elavil
- Pamelor

- Paxil
- BuSpar
- Lithium
- Serax
- Tofranil

Neuroleptics:

- Thorazine
- Haldol
- Zyprexa

Sedatives:

- Librium
- barbiturates

- Valium
- Ativan

- Xanax

Antihistamines: Associated with lack of lubrication in women leading to dyspareunia. In men, erectile dysfunction and decreased libido. Commonly used medications are:

- Dramamine
- Antivert

- Benadryl
- Phenergan

- Vistaril

Anticonvulsants: Associated with decreased libido, decreased arousal and orgasmic disorder in women and erectile dysfunction and decreased libido in men. Commonly used medications are:

- Dilantin
- Tegretol

- Mysoline
- Luminal

Medications used to treat gastric disorders: Associated with erectile dysfunction in men and decreased libido, decreased arousal and orgasmic disorder in women. Commonly used medications are:

- Tagamet
- Pepcid
  - Phenergan

- Reglan
- Compazine

- Zantac

Medications used to treat dyslipidemia: Associated with erectile dysfunction in men. Commonly used medications are the fibrates such as gemfibrozil.

Appendix A

Medications used to treat cancer: Associated with deceased libido and erectile dysfunction in men and dyspareunia in women. Commonly used medications are:

- Tamoxifen
- Nilutamide
- Ketoconazole
- Lupron
- Myleran
- Zoladex
- Flutamide
- Cytoxan
- Casodex

Birth control: Associated with decreased libido, arousal disorder and vaginal dryness in women. Commonly used medications are:

- Ortho 7/7/7
- Cyclen
- Tricyclen
- Depo Provera

Anti-Parkinson's: Associated with erectile dysfunction and increased libido in men and women. Commonly used medications are:

- Cogentin
- Sinemet
- Akineton
- Kemadrin
- Parlodel
- Artane

Non-steroidal anti-inflammatory: Associated with decreased lubrication. Commonly used medications are:

- Indocin
- Ibuprofen

Other medications: Associated with various sexual disorders. Commonly used medications are:

- Amicar
- Flexeril
- Proscar
- Atropine
- Lanoxin
- Propecia
- Compazine
- Norpace

Nonprescription drugs: Alcohol can cause decreased libido in men and women as well as orgasmic disorders and erectile dysfunction in men. Heroin and morphine can cause decreased libido in men and women and can cause ejaculatory disorders in men. Over time, amphetamines and cocaine can cause erectile dysfunction in men. Marijuana can cause vaginal dryness in women.

Appendix B

National Institutes of Health (NIH) Consensus Statement. Impotence. 1992.

Impotence, which affects about 30 million men in the United States, is the consistent inability to attain and maintain a penile erection sufficient to permit satisfactory sexual intercourse. An erection results from a complex interaction between muscles, nerves and blood vessels and is influenced by psychological and behavioral factors.

Men who see impotence as a natural consequence of aging may change their sexual expectations and behavior. Increasingly, however, men are seeking treatments to restore erectile function, while the medical community has not generally agreed on when to perform certain tests and offer specific treatments. Therefore, the National Institute of Diabetes and Digestive and Kidney Diseases and the NIH Office of Medical Applications of Research held a Consensus Development Conference on Impotence, December 7-9, 1992.

The panel of specialists in urology, nursing, endocrinology, cardiology gerontology, psychology, psychiatry, epidemiology, biostatistics and a representative of the general public arrived at the following conclusions.

Because the term impotence has significant negative overtones and has been used to describe a range of sexual problems, the panel favored using the specific term "erectile dysfunction."

The risk of erectile dysfunction increases with age, but men who have diabetes, hypertension, high cholesterol, low high-density lipoproteins, Peyronie's disease, priapism, depression, injuries or disorders affecting the nerves or blood, or who take prescription or other drugs are also at risk. Though cigarette smoking does not directly cause erectile dysfunction, it can increase the risk of vascular disease and hypertension.

Because erectile dysfunction is most often the result of a combination of psychological and physical factors, education about anxiety's role may help prevent or reduce the duration and severity of erectile dysfunction.

For men complaining of erectile dysfunction, the panel recommended a careful, detailed medical and sexual history, followed by a physical examination and basic laboratory studies to identify psychological factors as well as unrecognized disease.

The panel emphasized that a sexual history, an often neglected element of the evaluation, is vital to assess a man's true complaint, expectation, and motivation for further diagnosis and treatment. The sexual partner's perceptions should also be obtained if possible.

The physical examination should include the testicles, penis, prostate, anal sphincter tone, femoral and lower extremity pulses and neurologic examination of perianal sensation and bulbocavernosus reflex. Suspected neurological problems may require more extensive tests.

Laboratory studies should include a urinalysis and blood test for complete blood count, creatinine, lipid profile, fasting blood sugar, thyroid function and morning testosterone. Low testosterone indicates a second test for this hormone and luteinizing hormone and prolactin should also be measured.

The panel identified additional tests that might be useful in some men.

Nocturnal penile tumescence testing may be useful in men who report a complete absence of erections or when a primarily psychogenic cause is suspected.

Only men who are seriously considering penile injections, implants, or vascular surgery require intracavernous pharmacologic injection of a vasodilating agent to assess penile blood supply. If this test produces an erection, home penile injection therapy may be an option. However, anxiety or discomfort during the test may prevent an erection even in men who have adequate blood vessel function.

Duplex color ultrasonography, dynamic infusion pharmacocavernosometry and cavernosography and pharmacologic pelvic/penile angiography will further define vascular disorders to young men who do not respond to the penile injection test, do have a history of perineal or pelvic trauma and are serious candidates for vascular surgery. These tests are best done by experts in the vascular aspects of erectile dysfunction.

While the most common treatments—vacuum devices, injections and implants—are effective in producing erections in most men, many discontinue their use. Treatment may be more successful when the sexual partner participates in evaluation and when treatment, beginning with the least risky, is tailored to the couple's goals. Counseling is always recommended.

Hormone-related erectile dysfunction is relatively rare, but in cases of confirmed low serum testosterone, the panel recommended intramuscular injections of testosterone enanthate or cypionate. In cases of confirmed hyper- prolactinernia, the oral drug bromocryptine is appropriate. However, these treatments are inappropriate and may increase the risk of prostate cancer when testicular function is normal.

The panel found that while vacuum devices require manual dexterity, they are very effective in producing an erection and are relatively risk-free, although they may cause some discomfort and impair ejaculation.

The most effective agents for penile injection are papa- verine, phentolamine and prostaglandin El. They can be used in combination to reduce pain, penile corporal fibrosis, fibrotic nodules and priapism. Injections can be a problem for men who have poor vision, poor manual dexterity, psychiatric disease and for those who receive anticoagulant therapy or who cannot tolerate transient hypertension. In addition, drugs used to reverse priapism can cause death in men taking monoamine oxidase inhibitors for hypertension.

Mechanical failure, prostheses-associated infection (most common in men with diabetes, spinal cord injuries, or urinary tract infections) and erosion can occur with rigid, malleable, or inflatable penile prosthetics. Inflatable implants produce the most natural flaccid and erect states, but also have the highest failure and reoperation rates. No problems related to silicone migration from these implants have been reported.

The panel recommended that vascular surgery, which is often unsuccessful, be done only in a clinical research setting on young men who have congenital vascular defects or who have had pelvic or penile injuries.

Because of widespread ignorance, misinformation and embarrassment about erectile dysfunction, the panel encouraged dissemination of information through the media, community and health organizations and called for required education in human sexuality for health professionals.

Finally, the panel encouraged a multi-disciplinary approach to future investigations and urged researchers to develop diagnostic and treatment outcome standards. They also recommended epidemiological studies; studies on the racial, cultural, ethnic and social perceptions and expectations of erectile function and dysfunction; studies to identify means to prevent erectile dysfunction; and clinical trials to assess and compare behavioral, mechanical, pharmacologic and surgical treatments.

This conference was cosponsored by the National Institute of Neurological Disorders and Stroke and the National Institute on Aging.

NIH Consensus Statement. Impotence. Volume 10, Number 4, December 7-9, 1992. National Institutes of Health, Office of the Director. Free copies may also be downloaded at http://consensus.nih.gov/1992/1992 Impotence091PDF.pdf.

Appendix C
Body Mass Index (BMI) Table

To use the table, find the appropriate height in the left-hand column labeled Height. Move across to a given weight. The number at the top of the column is the BMI at that height and weight. Pounds have been rounded off.

BMI	19	20	21	22	23	24	25	26	27	28	29	30	31	32	33	34	35	36	37	38	39	40	41	42	43	44	45	46	47	48	49	50	51	52	53	54
Height (inches.)															**Body Weight (pounds)**																					
58	91	96	100	105	110	115	119	124	129	134	138	143	148	153	158	162	167	172	177	181	186	191	196	201	205	210	215	220	224	229	234	239	244	248	253	258
59	94	99	104	109	114	119	124	128	133	138	143	148	153	158	163	168	173	178	183	188	193	198	203	208	212	217	222	227	232	237	242	247	252	257	262	267
60	97	102	107	112	118	123	128	133	138	143	148	153	158	163	168	174	179	184	189	194	199	204	209	215	220	225	230	235	240	245	250	255	261	266	271	276
61	100	106	111	116	122	127	132	137	143	148	153	158	164	169	174	180	185	190	195	201	206	211	217	222	227	232	238	243	248	254	259	264	269	275	280	285
62	104	109	115	120	126	131	136	142	147	153	158	164	169	175	180	186	191	196	202	207	213	218	224	229	235	240	246	251	256	262	267	273	278	284	289	295
63	107	113	118	124	130	135	141	146	152	158	163	169	175	180	186	191	197	203	208	214	220	225	231	237	242	248	254	259	265	270	278	282	287	293	299	304
64	110	116	122	128	134	140	145	151	157	163	169	174	180	186	192	197	204	209	215	221	227	232	238	244	250	256	262	267	273	279	285	291	296	302	308	314
65	114	120	126	132	138	144	150	156	162	168	174	180	186	192	198	204	210	216	222	228	234	240	246	252	258	264	270	276	282	288	294	300	306	312	318	324
66	118	124	130	136	142	148	155	161	167	173	179	186	192	198	204	210	216	223	229	235	241	247	253	260	266	272	278	284	291	297	303	309	315	322	328	334
67	121	127	134	140	146	153	159	166	172	178	185	191	198	204	211	217	223	230	236	242	249	255	261	268	274	280	287	293	299	306	312	319	325	331	338	344
68	125	131	138	144	151	158	164	171	177	184	190	197	203	210	216	223	230	236	243	249	256	262	269	276	282	289	295	302	308	315	322	328	335	341	348	354
69	128	135	142	149	155	162	169	176	182	189	196	203	209	216	223	230	236	243	250	257	263	270	277	284	291	297	304	311	318	324	331	338	345	351	358	365
70	132	139	146	153	160	167	174	181	188	195	202	209	216	222	229	236	243	250	257	264	271	278	285	292	299	306	313	320	327	334	341	348	355	362	369	376
71	136	143	150	157	165	172	179	186	193	200	208	215	222	229	236	243	250	257	265	272	279	286	293	301	308	315	322	329	338	343	351	358	365	372	379	386
72	140	147	154	162	169	177	184	191	199	206	213	221	228	235	242	250	258	265	272	279	287	294	302	309	316	324	331	338	346	353	361	368	375	383	390	397
73	144	151	159	166	174	182	189	197	204	212	219	227	235	242	250	257	265	272	280	288	295	302	310	318	325	333	340	348	355	363	371	378	386	393	401	408
74	148	155	163	171	179	186	194	202	210	218	225	233	241	249	256	264	272	280	287	295	303	311	319	326	334	342	350	358	365	373	381	389	396	404	412	420
75	152	160	168	176	184	192	200	208	216	224	232	240	248	256	264	272	279	287	295	303	311	319	327	335	343	351	359	367	375	383	391	399	407	415	423	431
76	156	164	172	180	189	197	205	213	221	230	238	246	254	263	271	279	287	295	304	312	320	328	336	344	353	361	369	377	385	394	402	410	418	426	435	443

Source: National Heart, Lung and Blood Institute. National Institutes of Health http://www.nhlbi.nih.gov/guidelines/obesity/bmi_tbl.pdf

Appendix D

General Physical Activities Defined by Level of Intensity

The table below is in accordance with Centers for Disease Control and Prevention (CDC) and the American College of Sports Medicine (ACSM) guidelines.

MODERATE ACTIVITY+ 3.0 to 6.0 METs* (3.5 to 7 kcal/min)	VIGOROUS ACTIVITY+ Greater than 6.0 METs* (more than 7 kcal/min)
Walking at a moderate or brisk pace of 3 to 4.5 mph on a level surface inside or outside, such as • Walking to class, work, or the store; • Walking for pleasure; • Walking the dog; or • Walking as a break from work. • Walking downstairs or down a hill • Racewalking—less than 5 mph • Using crutches • Hiking • Roller skating or In-line skating at a leisurely pace	Racewalking and aerobic walking—5 mph or faster • Jogging or running • Wheeling your wheelchair • Walking and climbing briskly up a hill • Backpacking • Mountain climbing, rock climbing, rappelling • Roller skating or in-line skating at a brisk pace
• Bicycling 5 to 9 mph, level terrain, or with few hills • Stationary bicycling—using moderate effort	• Bicycling more than 10 mph or bicycling on steep uphill terrain • Stationary bicycling—using vigorous effort

MODERATE ACTIVITY+ 3.0 to 6.0 METs* (3.5 to 7 kcal/min)	VIGOROUS ACTIVITY+ Greater than 6.0 METs* (more than 7 kcal/min)
• Aerobic dancing—high impact • Water aerobics	• Aerobic dancing—high impact • Step aerobics • Water jogging • Teaching an aerobic dance class
• Calisthenics—light • Yoga • Gymnastics • General home exercises, light or moderate • Effort, getting up and down from the floor • Jumping on a trampoline • Using a stair climber machine at a light-to-moderate pace • Using a rowing machine—with moderate effort	• Calisthenics—push-ups, pull-ups, vigorous effort • Karate, judo, tae kwon do, jujitsu • Jumping rope • Performing jumping jacks • Using a stair climber machine at a fast pace • Using a rowing machine—with vigorous effort • Using an arm cycling machine—with vigorous effort
Weight training and bodybuilding using free weights, Nautilus- or Universal-type weights	Circuit weight training
• Boxing—punching bag	• Boxing—in the ring, sparring • Wrestling—competitive
• Ballroom dancing • Line dancing • Square dancing • Folk dancing • Modern dancing, disco • Ballet	• Professional ballroom dancing—energetically • Square dancing—energetically • Folk dancing—energetically • Clogging
• Table tennis—competitive • Tennis—doubles	• Tennis—singles • Wheelchair tennis
• Golf, wheeling or carrying clubs	• ——

MODERATE ACTIVITY+ 3.0 to 6.0 METs* (3.5 to 7 kcal/min)	VIGOROUS ACTIVITY+ Greater than 6.0 METs* (more than 7 kcal/min)
• Softball—fast pitch or slow pitch • Basketball—shooting baskets • Coaching children's or adults' sports	• Most competitive sports • Football game • Basketball game • Wheelchair basketball • Soccer • Rugby • Kickball • Field or rollerblade hockey • Lacrosse
• Volleyball—competitive • Playing Frisbee • Juggling • Curling • Cricket—batting and bowling • Badminton • Archery (nonhunting) • Fencing	• Beach volleyball—on sand court • Handball—general or team • Racquetball • Squash
• Downhill skiing—with light effort • Ice skating at a leisurely pace (9 mph or less) • Snowmobiling • Ice sailing	• Downhill skiing—racing or with vigorous effort • Ice-skating—fast pace or speedskating cross-country skiing • Sledding • Tobogganing • Playing ice hockey
• Swimming—recreational • Treading water—slowly, moderate effort • Diving—springboard or platform • Aquatic aerobics • Waterskiing • Snorkeling • Surfing, board or body	• Swimming—steady paced laps • Synchronized swimming • Treading water—fast, vigorous effort • Water jogging • Water polo • Water basketball • Scuba diving

MODERATE ACTIVITY+ 3.0 to 6.0 METs* (3.5 to 7 kcal/min)	VIGOROUS ACTIVITY+ Greater than 6.0 METs* (more than 7 kcal/min)
• Canoeing or rowing a boat at less than 4 mph • Rafting—whitewater • Sailing—recreational or competition • Paddle boating • Kayaking—on a lake, calm water • Washing or waxing a powerboat or the hull of a sailboat	• Canoeing or rowing—4 or more mph • Kayaking in whitewater rapids
• Fishing while walking along a riverbank or while wading in a stream—wearing waders	• ——
• Hunting deer, large or small game • Pheasant and goose hunting • Hunting with a bow and arrow or crossbow—walking	• ——
• Horseback riding—general saddling or grooming a horse	• Horseback riding—trotting, galloping, jumping, or in competition • Playing polo
• Playing on school playground equipment, moving about, swinging, or climbing • Playing hopscotch, 4-square, dodgeball, T-ball, or tetherball • Skateboarding • Roller-skating or In-line skating—leisurely pace	• Running • Skipping • Jumping rope • Performing jumping jacks • Roller-skating or in-line skating—fast pace
• Playing instruments while actively moving; playing in a marching band; playing guitar or drums in a rock band • Twirling a baton In a marching band • Singing while actively moving about—as on stage or In church	• Playing a heavy musical Instrument while actively running In a marching band

156

Appendix D

MODERATE ACTIVITY+ 3.0 to 6.0 METs* (3.5 to 7 kcal/min)	VIGOROUS ACTIVITY+ Greater than 6.0 METs* (more than 7 kcal/min)
• Gardening and yard work: raking the lawn, bagging grass or leaves, digging, hoeing, light shoveling (less than 10 lbs per minute), or weeding while standing or bending • Planting trees, trimming shrubs and trees, hauling branches, stacking wood • Pushing a power lawn mower or tiller	• Gardening and yard work: heavy or rapid shoveling (more than 10 lbs per minute), digging ditches, or carrying heavy loads • Felling trees, carrying large logs, swinging an ax, hand-splitting logs, or climbing and trimming trees • Pushing a non-motorized lawn mower
• Shoveling heavy snow	• Shoveling light snow
• Moderate housework: scrubbing the floor or bathtub while on hands and knees, hanging laundry on a clothesline, sweeping an outdoor area, cleaning out the garage, washing windows, moving light furniture, packing or unpacking boxes, walking and putting household items away, carrying out heavy bags of trash or recyclables (e.g., glass, newspapers and plastics), or carrying water or firewood • General household tasks requiring considerable effort	• Heavy housework: moving or pushing heavy furniture (75 lbs or more), carrying household items weighing 25 lbs or more up a flight or stairs, or shoveling coal into a stove • Standing, walking, or walking down a flight of stairs while carrying objects weighing 50 lbs or more
• Putting groceries away—walking and carrying especially large or heavy items less than 50 lbs.	• Carrying several heavy bags (25 lbs or more) of groceries at one time up a flight of stairs • Grocery shopping while carrying young children *and* pushing a full grocery cart, or pushing two full grocery carts at once
• Actively playing with children—walking, running, or climbing while playing with children • Walking while carrying a child weighing less than 50 lbs • Walking while pushing or pulling a child In a stroller or an adult In a wheelchair • Carrying a child weighing less than 25 lbs up a flight of stairs • Child care: handling uncooperative young children (e.g., chasing, dressing, lifting into car seat), or handling several young children at one time • Bathing and dressing an adult	• Vigorously playing with children—running longer distances or playing strenuous games with children • Racewalking or jogging while pushing a stroller designed for sport use • Carrying an adult or a child weighing 25 lbs or more up a flight of stairs • Standing or walking while carrying an adult or a child weighing 50 lbs or more

157

MODERATE ACTIVITY+ 3.0 to 6.0 METs* (3.5 to 7 kcal/min)	VIGOROUS ACTIVITY+ Greater than 6.0 METs* (more than 7 kcal/min)
• Animal care: shoveling grain, feeding farm animals, or grooming animals • Playing with or training animals • Manually milking cows or hooking cows up to milking machines	• Animal care: forking bales of hay or straw, cleaning a barn or stables, or carrying animals weighing over 50 lbs • Handling or carrying heavy animal related equipment or tack
• Home repair: cleaning gutters, caulking, refinishing furniture, sanding floors with a power sander, or laying or removing carpet or tiles • General home construction work: roofing, painting inside or outside of the house, wall papering, scraping, plastering, or remodeling	• Home repair or construction: very hard physical labor, standing or walking while carrying heavy loads of 50 lbs or more, taking loads of 25 lbs or more up a flight of stairs or ladder (e.g., carrying roofing materials onto the roof), or concrete or masonry work
• Outdoor carpentry, sawing wood with a power saw	• Hand-sawing hardwoods
• Automobile bodywork • Hand washing and waxing a car	• Pushing a disabled car

MODERATE ACTIVITY+ 3.0 to 6.0 METs* (3.5 to 7 kcal/min)	VIGOROUS ACTIVITY+ Greater than 6.0 METs* (more than 7 kcal/min)
• Occupations that require extended periods of walking, pushing or pulling objects weighing less than 75 lbs, standing while lifting objects less than 50 lbs or carrying objects of less than 25 lbs up a flight of stairs. • Tasks frequently requiring moderate effort and considerable use of arms, legs or occasional total body movements. For example: • Briskly walking on a level surface while carrying a suitcase or load weighing up to 50 lbs • Maid service or cleaning services • Waiting tables or institutional dishwashing • Driving or maneuvering heavy vehicles (e.g., semi-truck, school bus, tractor or harvester)—not fully automated and requiring extensive use of arms and legs • Operating heavy power tools (e.g., drills and jackhammers) • Many homebuilding tasks (e.g., electrical work, plumbing, carpentry, dry wall and painting) • Farming—feeding and grooming animals, milking cows, shoveling grain, picking fruit from trees or picking vegetables • Packing boxes for shipping or moving • Assembly-line work—tasks requiring movement of the entire body, arms or legs with moderate effort • Mail carriers—walking while carrying a mailbag • Patient care—bathing, dressing and moving patients or physical therapy	• Occupations that require extensive periods of running, rapid movement, pushing or pulling objects weighing 75 lbs or more, standing while lifting heavy objects of 50 pounds or more, walking while carrying heavy objects of 25 lbs or more. • Tasks frequently requiring strenuous effort and extensive total body movements. For example: • Running up a flight of stairs while carrying a suitcase or load weighing 25 lbs or more • Teaching a class or skill requiring active and strenuous participation, such as aerobics or physical education instructor • Firefighting • Masonry or heavy construction work • Coal mining • Manually shoveling or digging ditches • Using heavy non-powered tools • Most forestry work • Farming—forking straw, baling hay, cleaning barn, or poultry work • Moving items professionally • Loading or unloading a truck

Source: U.S. Department of Health and Human Services, Public Health Service, Centers for Disease Control and Prevention, National Center for Chronic Disease Prevention and Health Promotion, Division of Nutrition and Physical Activity. *Promoting physical activity: a guide for community action*. Champaign, IL: Human Kinetics, 1999. Web site: http://www.cdc.gov/nccdphp/dnpa/physical/pdf/PA_Intensity_table_2_1.pdf
(Table adapted from Ainsworth BE, Haskell WL, Leon AS, et al. Compendium of physical activities: classification of energy costs of human physical activities. *Medicine and Science in Sports and Exercise* 1993; 25(I):71 80. Adapted with technical assistance from Dr. Barbara Ainsworth.)

- *The ratio of exercise metabolic rate. One MET is defined as the energy expenditure for sitting quietly, which, for the average adult, approximates 3.5 ml of oxygen uptake per kilogram of body weight per minute (1.2 kcal/min for a 70 kg individual). For example, a 2 MET activity requires two times the metabolic energy expenditure of sitting quietly.
- +For an average person, defined here as 70 kilograms or 154 pounds. The activity intensity levels, portrayed in this chart are most applicable to men aged 30 to 50 years and women aged 20 to 40 years. For older individuals, the classification of activity intensity might be higher. For example, what is moderate intensity to a 40-year-old man might be vigorous for a man in his 70s. Intensity is a subjective classification.

Data for this chart were available only for adults. Therefore, when children's games are listed, the estimated intensity level is for adults participating in children's activities. To compute the amount of time needed to accumulate 150 kcal, do the following calculation: 150 kcal divided by the MET level of the activity equals the minutes needed to expend 150 kcal. For example: 150 +3 METS = 50 minutes of participation. Generally, activities in the *moderate* intensity range require 25 to 50 minutes to expend a moderate amount of activity and activities in the *vigorous* intensity range would require less than 25 minutes to achieve a moderate amount of activity. Each activity listed is categorized as light, moderate, or vigorous on the basis of current knowledge of the overall level of intensity required for the average person to engage in it, taking into account brief periods when the level of intensity required for the activity might increase or decrease considerably.

Persons with disabilities, including motor function limitations (e.g., quadriplegia), may wish to consult with an exercise physiologist or physical therapist to properly classify the types of physical activities in which they might participate, including assisted exercise. Certain activities classified in this listing as *moderate* might be *vigorous* for persons who must overcome physical challenges or disabilities.

Note: Almost every occupation requires some mix of light, moderate, or vigorous activities, depending on the task at hand. To categorize the activity level of your own position, ask yourself: How many minutes each working day do I spend doing the types of activities described as light, moderate, or vigorous?

To arrive at a total workday caloric expenditure, multiply the minutes spent doing activities within each intensity level by the kilocalories corresponding to each level of intensity. Then, add together the total kilocalories spent doing light, moderate and vigorous activities to arrive at your total energy expenditure in a typical day.

Appendix E

Risk from Sexual Activity in Cardiovascular Diseases

Low risk. Typically implied by the ability to perform exercise of modest intensity without symptoms.

Asymptomatic and <3 major risk factors (excluding gender)

Major cardiovascular disease risk factors include age, male gender, hypertension, diabetes mellitus, cigarette smoking, dyslipidemia, sedentary lifestyle and family history of premature CAD

Controlled hypertension

Beta blockers and thiazide diuretics may predispose to ED

Mild, stable angina pectoris

Noninvasive evaluation recommended

Antianginal drug regimen may require modification

Postrevascularization and without significant residual ischemia

ETT may be beneficial to assess risk

Post-myocardial infarction (MI) (>6-8 weeks), but asymptomatic and without ETT-induced ischemia, or postrevascularization.

If postrevascularization or no ETT-induced ischemia, intercourse may be resumed 3-4 weeks post-MI

Mild valvular disease

May include select patients with mild aortic stenosis

LVD (NYHA class 1)

Most patients are low risk

Intermediate or indeterminate risk. Evaluate to reclassify as high or low risk.

Asymptomatic and CAD risk factors (excluding gender)
 Increased risk for acute MI and death
 ETT may be appropriate, particularly in sedentary patients
Moderate, stable angina pectoris
 ETT may clarify risk
MI >2 weeks but <6 weeks
 Increased risk of ischemia, reinfarction and malignant arrhythmias
 ETT may clarify risk
LVD/congestive heart failure (CHF) (NYHA class 11)
 Moderate risk of increased symptoms
 Cardiovascular evaluation and rehabilitation may permit reclassification as low risk
Noncardiac atherosclerotic sequelae (peripheral arterial disease, history of stroke, or transient ischemic attacks)
 Increased risk of MI
 Cardiological evaluation should be considered

High Risk. Defer resumption of sexual activity until cardiological assessment and treatment.

Unstable or refractory angina
 Increased risk of MI
Uncontrolled hypertension
 Increased risk of acute cardiac and vascular events (i.e., stroke)
CHF (NYHA class 111, IV)
 Increased risk of cardiac decompensation
Recent MI (<2 weeks)
 Increased risk of reinfarction, cardiac rupture, or arrhythmias, but impact of complete revascularization on risk is unknown
High-risk arrhythmias
 Rarely, malignant arrhythmias during sexual activity may cause sudden death
 Risk is decreased by an implanted defibrillator or pacemaker
Obstructive hypertrophic cardiomyopathies
 Cardiovascular risks of sexual activity are poorly defined

Cardiological evaluation (i.e., exercise stress testing and echocardiography) may guide patient management
Moderate to severe valve disease
Use vasoactive drugs with caution

CAD = coronary artery disease;
CHIF = congestive heart failure;
CV = cardio vascular;
CVA = cerebrovascular accident;
ED = erectile dysfunction;
ETT exercise tolerance test;
WD = left ventricular dysfunction;
MI = myocardial infarction;
NYHA = New York Heart Association.

Adapted from: Kostis JB et al. Sexual dysfunction and cardiac risk (the Second Princeton Consensus Conference). *Am J Cardiol.* 2005 Jul 15; 96(2):313-21.

Appendix F

International Index of Erectile Function (IIEF) Questionnaire

Date of visit:_____

Please use an X where applicable and be sure to initial and date all corrections.

Score 0 if not done   Subject questionnaire - Section 1

Instructions: These questions ask about the effects your erection problems have had on your sex life, *over the past 4 weeks*. Please answer the following questions as honestly and clearly as possible. In answering these questions, the following definitions apply:

Definitions:

Sexual activity includes intercourse, caressing, foreplay and masturbation

Sexual intercourse is defined as vaginal penetration of the partner (you entered the partner)

Sexual stimulation includes situations like foreplay with a partner, looking at erotic pictures, etc.

Ejaculate is defined as the ejection of semen from the penis (or the feeling of this)

Mark only one answer per question.

1. Over the past 4 weeks, how often were you able to get an erection during sexual activity?

0   No sexual activity
1   Almost never or never
2   A few times (much less than half the time)
3   Sometimes (about half the time)
4   Most times (much more than half the time)
5   Almost always or always

2. Over the past 4 weeks, when you had erections with sexual stimulation, how often were your erections hard enough for penetration?

0   No sexual stimulation
1   Almost never or never
2   A few times (much less than half the time)
3   Sometimes (about half the time)
4   Most times (much more than half the time)
5   Almost always or always

Questions 3, 4 and 5 will ask about erections you may have had during sexual intercourse.

3. Over the past 4 weeks, when you attempted sexual intercourse, how often were you able to penetrate (enter) your partner?

0   No sexual activity
1   Almost never or never
2   A few times (much less than half the time)
3   Sometimes (about half the time)
4   Most times (much more than half the time)
5   Almost always or always

4. Over the past 4 weeks, during sexual intercourse, how often were you able to maintain your erection after you had penetrated (entered) your partner?

   0   No sexual activity
   1   Almost never or never
   2   A few times (much less than half the time)
   3   Sometimes (about half the time)
   4   Most times (much more than half the time)
   5   Almost always or always

5. Over the past 4 weeks, during sexual intercourse, how difficult was it to maintain your erection to completion of intercourse?

   0   No sexual activity
   1   Extremely difficult
   2   Very difficult
   3   Difficult
   4   Slightly difficult
   5   Not difficult

6. Over the past 4 weeks, how many times have you attempted sexual intercourse?

   0   No attempts
   1   1-2 attempts
   2   3-4 attempts
   3   5-6 attempts
   4   7-10 attempts
   5   11 or more attempts

7. Over the past 4 weeks, when you attempted sexual intercourse how often was it satisfactory for you?

   0   No sexual activity
   1   Almost never or never
   2   A few times (much less than half the time)
   3   Sometimes (about half the time)
   4   Most times (much more than half the time)
   5   Almost always or always

8. Over the past 4 weeks, how much have you enjoyed sexual intercourse?

    0   No intercourse
    1   Not enjoyable
    2   Not very enjoyable
    3   Fairly enjoyable
    4   Highly enjoyable
    5   Very highly enjoyable

9. Over the past 4 weeks, when you had sexual stimulation or intercourse how often did you ejaculate?

    0   No sexual activity
    1   Almost never
    2   A few times (much less than half the time)
    3   Sometimes (about half the time)
    4   Most times (much more than half the time)
    5   Almost always or always

10. Over the past 4 weeks, when you had sexual stimulation or intercourse how often did you have the feeling of orgasm or climax (with or without ejaculation)?

    0   No sexual activity
    1   Almost never
    2   A few times (much less than half the time)
    3   Sometimes (about half the time)
    4   Most times (much more than half the time)
    5   Almost always or always

Questions 11 and 12 ask about sexual desire. Let's define sexual desire as a feeling that may include wanting to have a sexual experience (for example, masturbation or intercourse), thinking about having sex or feeling frustrated due to a lack of sex.

11. Over the past 4 weeks, how often have you felt sexual desire?

0   No sexual activity
1   Almost never
2   A few times (much less than half the time)
3   Sometimes (about half the time)
4   Most times (much more than half the time)
5   Almost always or always

12. Over the past 4 weeks, how would you rate your level of sexual *desire?*

1   Very low or none at all
2   Low
3   Moderate
4   High
5   Very high

13. Over the past 4 weeks, how satisfied have you been with your overall *sex life?*

1   Very dissatisfied
2   Moderately dissatisfied
3   About equally satisfied and dissatisfied
4   Moderately satisfied
5   Very satisfied

14. Over the past 4 weeks, how satisfied have you been with your *sexual relationship* with your partner?

1   Very dissatisfied
2   Moderately dissatisfied
3   About equally satisfied and dissatisfied
4   Moderately satisfied
5   Very satisfied

15. Over the past 4 weeks, how do you rate your confidence that you can get and keep your erection?

1 Very low
2 Low
3 Moderate
4 High
1 Very high

Scoring for International Index of Erectile Function (IIEF) Questionnaire

All items are scored in 5 domains as follows:

Domain	Items	Range	Score Max Score
Erectile Function	1, 2, 3, 4, 5, 15	0-5	30
Orgasmic Function	9, 10	0-5	10
Sexual Desire	11, 12	1-5	10 15
Intercourse Satisfaction	6, 7, 8	0-5	15
Overall Satisfaction	13, 14, 10	1-5	10

Clinical Interpretation

I.   Erectile function total scores can be interpreted as follows:

Score	Interpretation
0-6	Severe dysfunction
7-12	Moderate dysfunction
13-18	Mild-to-moderate dysfunction
19-24	Mild dysfunction
25-30	No dysfunction

II.   Orgasmic function total scores can be interpreted as follows:

Score	Interpretation
0-2	Severe dysfunction
3-4	Moderate dysfunction
5-6	Mild-to-moderate dysfunction

Score	Interpretation
0-2	Severe dysfunction
7-8	Mild dysfunction
9-10	No dysfunction

III. Sexual desire total scores can be interpreted as follows:

Score	Interpretation
0-2	Severe dysfunction
3-4	Moderate dysfunction
5-6	Mild-to-moderate dysfunction
7-8	Mild dysfunction
9-10	No dysfunction

IV. Intercourse satisfaction total scores can be interpreted as follows:

Score	Interpretation
0-3	Severe dysfunction
4-6	Moderate dysfunction
7-9	Mild-to-moderate dysfunction
10-12	Mild dysfunction
13-15	No dysfunction

V. Overall satisfaction total scores can be interpreted as follows:

Score	Interpretation
0-2	Severe dysfunction
3-4	Moderate dysfunction
5-6	Mild-to-moderate dysfunction
7-8	Mild dysfunction
9-10	No dysfunction

Source: Rosen RC, Riley A, Wagner G, Osterloh IH, Kirkpatrick J, Mishra A. The international index of erectile function (IIEF) a multidimensional scale for assessment of erectile dysfunction. *Urology.* 1997 Jun; 49(6):822-30. Copyright 1997 by Elsevier Science, Inc.

Appendix G

American Urological Association Symptom Index for Benign Prostatic Hyperplasia Questionnaire

1. Over the last month or so, how often have you had a sensation of not emptying your bladder completely after you finished urinating?

0   Not at all
1   Less than 1 time in 5
2   Less than ½ the time
3   About ½ the time
4   More than ½ the time
5   Almost always

2. During the last month or so, how often have you had to urinate again less than two hours after you finished urinating?

0   Not at all
1   Less than 1 time in 5
2   Less than ½ the time
3   About ½ the time
4   More than ½ the time
5   Almost always

3. During the last month or so, how often have you stopped and started again several times when you urinated?

   0   Not at all
   1   Less than 1 time in 5
   2   Less than ½ the time
   3   About ½ the time
   4   More than ½ the time
   5   Almost always

4. During the last month or so, how often have you found it difficult to postpone urination?

   0   Not at all
   1   Less than 1 time in 5
   2   Less than ½ the time
   3   About ½ the time
   4   More than ½ the time
   5   Almost always

5. During the last month or so, how often have you had a weak urinary stream?

   0   Not at all
   1   Less than 1 time in 5
   2   Less than ½ the time
   3   About ½ the time
   4   More than ½ the time
   5   Almost always

6. During the last month or so, how often have you had to push or strain to begin urination?

   0   Not at all
   1   Less than 1 time in 5
   2   Less than ½ the time
   3   About ½ the time
   4   More than ½ the time
   5   Almost always

7. During the last month, how many times did you most typically get up to urinate from the time you went to bed at night until the time you got up in the morning?

0 None
1 1 time
2 2 times
3 3 times
4 4 times
5 5 or more times

Add the score for each number above.

Symptom Score	
1-7	Mild
8-19	Moderate
20-35	Severe

Quality of Life

How would you feel if you had to live with your urinary condition the way it is now, no better, no worse, for the rest of your life?

0 Delighted
1 Pleased
2 Mostly satisfied
3 Mixed
4 Mostly dissatisfied
5 Unhappy
6 Terrible

Source: Adapted from Barry MJ, Fowler FJ Jr, O'Leary MP, Bruskewitz RC, Holtgrewe HL, Mebust WK, Cockett AT. The American Urological Association symptom index for benign prostatic hyperplasia. The Measurement Committee of the American Urological Association. *J Urol*. 1992 Nov; 148(5):1549-57; discussion 1564. Copyright 1992 American Urological Association.

Appendix H

Sexual Health Inventory for Men (SHIM) Questionnaire

Each question has several possible responses. Circle the number of the response that best describes your own situation. Please be sure that you select one and only one for each question.

Over the Past Six Months:

1. How do you rate your confidence that you could get and keep an erection?

None	Very Low	Low	Moderate	High	Very High
0	1	2	3	4	5

2. When you had erections with sexual stimulation, how often were your erections hard enough for penetration (entering your partner)?

No sexual activity	Almost never or never	A few times (much less than ½ the time)	Sometimes (about ½ the time)	Most times (much more than ½ the time)	Almost always or always
0	1	2	3	4	5

3. During sexual intercourse, how often were you able to maintain your erection after you had penetrated (entered) your partner?

Did not attempt intercourse	Almost never or never	A few times (much less than ½ the time)	Sometimes (about ½ the time)	Most times (much more than ½ the time)	Almost always or always
0	1	2	3	4	5

4. During sexual intercourse, how difficult was it to maintain your erection to completion of intercourse?

Did not attempt intercourse	Extremely difficult	Very difficult	Difficult	Slightly difficult	Not difficult
0	1	2	3	4	5

5. When you attempted sexual intercourse, how often was it satisfactory for you?

Did not attempt intercourse	Almost never or never	A few times (much less than ½ the time)	Sometimes (about ½ the time)	Most times (much more than ½ the time)	Almost always or always
0	1	2	3	4	5

KEY

22-25	Normal erectile function
17-21	Mild ED
12-16	Mild to moderate ED
8-11	Moderate ED
≤7	Severe ED

Name: _____

Score: _____

Appendix I

Female Sexual Function Index (FSFI) Questionnaire

1. Over the past four weeks, how often did you feel sexual desire or interest?

5   Almost always or always
4   Most times (more often than half the time)
3   Sometimes (about half the time)
2   A few times (less than half the time)
1   Almost never or never

2. Over the past four weeks, how would you rate your level (degree) of sexual desire or interest?

5   Very high
4   High
3   Moderate
2   Low
1   Very low or none at all

3. Over the past four weeks, how often did you feel sexually aroused ("turned on") during sexual activity or intercourse?

    0   No sexual activity
    5   Almost always or always
    4   Most times (more than half the time)
    3   Sometimes (about half the time)
    2   A few times (less than half the time)
    1   Almost never or never

4. Over the past four weeks, how would you rate your level of sexual arousal ("turn on") during sexual activity or intercourse?

    0   No sexual activity
    5   Very high
    4   High
    3   Moderate
    2   Low
    1   Very low or none at all

5. Over the past four weeks, how confident were you about becoming sexually aroused during sexual activity or intercourse?

    0   No sexual activity
    5   Very high confidence
    4   High confidence
    3   Moderate confidence
    2   Low confidence
    1   Very low or no confidence

6. Over the past four weeks, how often have you been satisfied with your arousal (excitement) during sexual activity or intercourse?

    0   No sexual activity
    5   Almost always or always
    4   Most times (more than half the time)
    3   Sometimes (about half the time)
    2   A few times (less than half the time)
    1   Almost never or never

7. Over the past four weeks, how often did you become lubricated ("wet") during sexual activity or intercourse?

    0   No sexual activity
    5   Almost always or always
    4   Most times (more than half the time)
    3   Sometimes (about half the time)
    2   A few times (less than half the time)
    1   Almost never or never

8. Over the past four weeks, how difficult was it to become lubricated ("wet") during sexual activity or intercourse?

    0   No sexual activity
    1   Extremely difficult or impossible
    2   Very difficult
    3   Difficult
    4   Slightly difficult
    5   Not difficult

9. Over the past four weeks, how often did you maintain your lubrication ("wetness") until completion of sexual activity or intercourse?

    0   No sexual activity
    5   Almost always or always
    4   Most times (more than half the time)
    3   Sometimes (about half the time)
    2   A few times (less than half the time)
    1   Almost never or never

10. Over the past four weeks, how difficult was it to maintain your lubrication (wetness) until completion of sexual activity or intercourse?

    0   No sexual activity
    1   Extremely difficult
    2   Very difficult
    3   Difficult
    4   Slightly difficult
    5   Not difficult

11. Over the past four weeks, when you had sexual stimulation or intercourse, how often did you reach orgasm (climax)?

0 No sexual activity
5 Almost always or always
4 Most times (more than half the time)
3 Sometimes (about half the time)
2 A few times (less than half the time)
1 Almost never or never

12. Over the past four weeks, when you had sexual stimulation or intercourse, how difficult was it for you to reach orgasm (climax)?

0 No sexual activity
1 Extremely difficult
2 Very difficult
3 Difficult
4 Slightly difficult
5 Not difficult

13. Over the past four weeks, how satisfied were you with your ability to reach orgasm (climax) during sexual activity or intercourse?

0 No sexual activity
5 Very satisfied
4 Moderately satisfied
3 About equally satisfied and dissatisfied
2 Moderately dissatisfied
1 Very dissatisfied

14. Over the past four weeks, how satisfied have you been with the amount of emotional closeness during sexual activity between you and your partner?

0 No sexual activity
5 Very satisfied
4 Moderately satisfied
3 About equally satisfied and dissatisfied
2 Moderately dissatisfied
1 Very dissatisfied

Sex and the Heart

15. Over the past four weeks, how satisfied have you been with your sexual relationship with your partner?

5   Very satisfied
4   Moderately satisfied
3   About equally satisfied and dissatisfied
2   Moderately dissatisfied
1   Very dissatisfied

16. Over the past four weeks, how satisfied have you been with your overall sexual life?

5   Very satisfied
4   Moderately satisfied
3   About equally satisfied and dissatisfied
2   Moderately dissatisfied
1   Very dissatisfied

17. Over the past four weeks, how often did you experience discomfort or pain during vaginal penetration?

0   Did not attempt intercourse
1   Almost always or always
2   Most times (more than half the time)
3   Sometimes (about half the time)
4   A few times (less than half the time)
5   Almost never or never

18. Over the past four weeks, how often did you experience discomfort or pain following vaginal penetration?

0   Did not attempt intercourse
1   Almost always or always
2   Most times (more than half the time)
3   Sometimes (about half the time)
4   A few times (less than half the time)
5   Almost never or never

19. Over the past four weeks, how would you rate your level (degree) of discomfort or pain during or following vaginal penetration?

    0   Did not attempt intercourse
    1   Very high
    2   High
    3   Moderate
    4   Low
    5   Very low or none at all

Scoring System:

The individual domain scores and full scale score of the FSFI are derived by the computational formula outlined in the table below. Individual domain scores are obtained by adding the scores of the individual items that comprise the domain and multiplying the sum by the domain factor (see below). The full scale score is obtained by adding the six domain scores. It should be noted that within the individual domains, a domain score of zero indicates that no sexual activity was reported during the past month.

Domain	Questions	Score Range	Factor	Minimum Score	Maximum Score	Score
Desire	1, 2	1-5	0.6	1.2	6.0	
Arousal	3,4,5,6	0-5	0.3	0	6.0	
Lubrication	7, 8, 9, 10	0-5	0.3	0	6.0	
Orgasm	11, 12, 13	0-5	0.4	0	6.0	
Satisfaction	14, 15, 16	0(Or 1)-5	0.4	0.8	6.0	
Pain	17, 18, 19	0-5	0.4	0	6.0	
Full Score Range		2.0	36.0			

Source: Rosen R, Brown C, Heiman J, Leiblum S, Meston C, Shabsigh R, Ferguson D, D'Agostino R Jr. The Female Sexual Function Index (FSFI): a multidimensional self-report instrument for the assessment of female sexual function. *J Sex Marital Ther.* 2000 Apr-Jun; 26(2):191-208. Copyright 2000 Brunner/Mazel.

Appendix J

Urological Information for Consumers

Northeast Indiana Urology, Fort Wayne, Indiana
  http://www.neiurology.com/

Sex and the Heart.org
  http://www.sexandtheheart.org

Seek Wellness Men's Sexuality Center
  http://www.seekwellness.com/mensexuality/

Seek Wellness Women's Sexuality Center
  http://www.seekwellness.com/womensexuality/

Consortium for Improvement in Erectile Function
  http://erectilefunction.org/

American Urological Association (AUA) patient information resource
  http://www.urologyhealth.org/

Urology channel—Erectile dysfunction
  http://www.urologychannel.com/erectiledysfunction/
  index.shtml

National Kidney and Urologic Diseases Information Clearinghouse
  (NKUDIC)
  http://www.kidney.niddk.nih.gov/

Health information from the National Library of Medicine and the
  National Institutes of Health http://www. Medlineplus.gov/

FamilyDoctor.org from the American Academy of Family Physicians
  http://familydoctor.org/

American Board of Medical Specialties
    http://www.abms.org

Dietary Guidelines for Americans
    US Department of Health and Human Services (HHS) and the
    Department of Agriculture (USDA)   http://www.health.gov/
    DietaryGuidelines/

Urological Information for Health Professionals

Sexual Medicine Society of North America, Inc.
    http://www.smsna.org/

American Urological Association (AUA)
    http://www.auanet.org/

AMS Medical Solutions
    http://www.americanmedicalsystems.com/

Mentor, a medical device company
    http://www.mentorcorp.com/

Medications for erectile dysfunction in men

Viagra®
    http://www.viagra.com/

Levitra®
    http://www.levitra.com/

Cialis®
    http://www.cialis.com/

Bibliography

1. Sex and exercise after a heart attack, Medical Online. http://www.medicalonline.com.au/medical/disease_index/hea rt/attack.htm
2. American Heart Association. Make healthy food choices. Http://www.americanheart.org/presenter .jhtml?identifier=537
3. American Heart Association. Delicious decisions: supermarket. Food label glossary & diagram. Http://www.delicious decisions.org/sm/fle_food_main.html
4. UCSB's SexInfo: Food sex drive boosters, University of California at Santa Barbara: Santa Barbara, CA. http://www.soc.ucsb.edu/sexinfo/print.php?article=faq&refid= 038
5. Aphrodisiac foods, GourmetSleuth.com. Http://www.gourmet sleuth.com/aphrodis_foods.htm
6. Discovery.com, Sexual Health Center. Aphrodisiacs, Discovery Communications, Inc. Http://www.health. Discovery.com/ centers/sex/aphrodisiacs/aphrodisiacs.html
7. Impotence. NIH Consensus Statement. 1992, National Institutes of Health: Washington, DC. p. 1-31. Http://consensus.nih.gov/ 1992/1992Impotence091PDF.pdf
8. General physical activities defined by level of intensity. In Centers for Disease Control and Prevention, National Center for Chronic Disease Prevention and Health Promotion, Division of Nutrition and Physical Activity. Promoting physical activity: a

guide for community action. 1999, Champaign, IL: Human Kinetics. 408.

9. American Heart Association. Scientific position: dietary guidelines for healthy American adults. 2000, American Heart Association: Dallas.

10. Sex and the heart: new guidelines for men. *Harv Mens Health Watch*, 2002. 6(10): 6-8.

11. Take pressure off your sex life. High blood pressure can contribute to sexual problems, as can some treatments for it. *Harv Heart Lett*, 2004. 15(2): 4.

12. Sexual and urologic problems of diabetes. National Diabetes Information Clearinghouse. NIH Publication No. 04–5135. 2004, National Institute of Diabetes and Digestive and Kidney Diseases (NIDDK): Washington, DC. Http://diabetes.niddk. nih.gov/dm/pubs/sup/index.htm

13. Dietary guidelines for Americans. 2005, Washington, DC: Department of Health and Human Services (HHS) and the Department of Agriculture (USDA). 84. Http://www. healthierus.gov/dietaryguidelines/

14. Role of age in erectile dysfunction examined, in *Daily Medical News*. 2005.

15. Exercise can spice up your sex life, the American Council on Exercise says. 2005, *Medical News Today*.

16. Survey of literature. *J Sex Med*, 2005. 2(2): 279-282.

17. Erectile dysfunction predictive of stroke in smokers, in *Daily Medical News*. 2006.

18. Althof, S.E., et al., Current perspectives on the clinical assessment and diagnosis of female sexual dysfunction and clinical studies of potential therapies: a statement of concern. *J Sex Med*, 2005. 2 Suppl 3: 146-53.

19. Althof, S.E., et al., Sildenafil citrate improves self-esteem, confidence, and relationships in men with erectile dysfunction: results from an international, multi-center, double-blind, placebo-controlled trial. *J Sex Med*, 2006. 3: 521-529.

20. Amsterdam, A., et al., Persistent sexual arousal syndrome associated with increased soy intake. *J Sex Med*, 2005. 2(3): 338-40.

21. Andersson, K.E., Erectile physiological and pathophysiological pathways involved in erectile dysfunction. *J Urol*, 2003. 170(2 Pt 2): S6-13; discussion S13-4.

22. Aronson, D., et al., C-Reactive protein is inversely related to physical fitness in middle-aged subjects. *Atherosclerosis*, 2004. 176(1): 173-9.

23. Arruda-Olson, A.M., et al., Cardiovascular effects of sildenafil during exercise in men with known or probable coronary artery disease: a randomized crossover trial. *JAMA*, 2002. 287(6): 719-25.

24. Bacon, C.G., et al., Sexual function in men older than 50 years of age: results from the health professionals follow-up study. *Ann Intern Med*, 2003. 139(3): 161-8.

25. Barrett-Connor, E., Cardiovascular risk stratification and cardiovascular risk factors associated with erectile dysfunction: assessing cardiovascular risk in men with erectile dysfunction. *Clin Cardiol*, 2004. 27(4 Suppl 1): 18-13.

26. Basson, R., et al., Summary of the recommendations on sexual dysfunctions in women. *J Sex Med*, 2004. 1(1): 24-34.

27. Basson, R., et al., Assessment and management of women's sexual dysfunctions: problematic desire and arousal. *J Sex Med*, 2005. 2(3): 291-300.

28. Beckley, E.T., Food for thought. DOC News, 2005. 2(3): 1-10.

29. Berman, J., L. Berman, and E. Bumiller, *For women only: a revolutionary guide to overcoming sexual dysfunction and reclaiming your sex life*. 2001, New York: Henry Holt and Company.

30. Berman, L., J. Berman, and A.B. Schweger, *Secrets of the sexually satisfied woman: ten keys to unlocking ultimate pleasure*. 2005, New York: Hyperion.

31. Billups, K.L., et al., Erectile dysfunction is a marker for cardiovascular disease: results of the minority health institute expert advisory panel. *J Sex Med*, 2005. 2(1): 40-50; discussion 50-2.

32. Block, J.D. and S.C. Bakos, *Sex over 50*. 1999, New York: Penguin Putnam Inc.

33. Bocchio, M., et al., Intima-media thickening of common carotid arteries is a risk factor for severe erectile dysfunction in men

with vascular risk factors but no clinical evidence of atherosclerosis. *J Urol*, 2005. 173(2): 526-9.

34. Bohlen, J.G., et al., Heart rate, rate-pressure product, and oxygen uptake during four sexual activities. *Arch Intern Med*, 1984. 144(9): 1745-8.

35. Boone, T. and S. Gilmore, Effects of sexual intercourse on maximal aerobic power, oxygen pulse, and double product in male sedentary subjects. *J Sports Med Phys Fitness*, 1995. 35(3): 214-7.

36. Braun, M., et al., Epidemiology of erectile dysfunction: results of the 'Cologne Male Survey'. *Int J Impot Res*, 2000. 12(6): 305-11.

37. Brawer, M.K., Androgen supplementation and prostate cancer risk: strategies for pretherapy assessment and monitoring. *Rev Urol*, 2003. 5 Suppl 1: S29-S33.

38. Brock, G.B., Issues in the assessment and treatment of erectile dysfunction: individualizing and optimizing therapy for the "silent majority," in *Medscape Today - CME*. 2002. http://www.medscape.com/viewprogram/1826

39. Bultrini, A., et al., Possible correlation between type 1 diabetes mellitus and female sexual dysfunction: case report and literature review. *J Sex Med*, 2004. 1(3): 337-40.

40. Burnett, A.L., Neuroprotection and nerve grafts in the treatment of neurogenic erectile dysfunction. *J Urol*, 2003. 170(2 Pt 2): S31-4; discussion S34.

41. Burnett, A.L., Widening the scope of erectile dysfunction risk associations. *J Urol*, 2005. 174(1): I2-3.

42. Calabro, P., et al., Release of C-reactive protein in response to inflammatory cytokines by human adipocytes: linking obesity to vascular inflammation. *J Am Coll Cardiol*, 2005. 46(6): 1112-3.

43. Cappelleri, J.C., et al., Comparison between sildenafil-treated subjects with erectile dysfunction and control subjects on the self-esteem and relationship questionnaire. *J Sex Med*, 2006. 3(2): 274-82.

44. Carani, C., et al., Multicenter study on the prevalence of sexual symptoms in male hypo- and hyperthyroid patients. *J Clin Endocrinol Metab*, 2005. 90(12): 6472-9.

45. Carruthers, M., Androgen deficiency in the adult male: causes, diagnosis and treatment. 2004, London: Taylor & Francis.

46. Carson, C.C., et al., Erectile response with vardenafil in sildenafil nonresponders: a multicenter, double-blind, 12-week, flexible-dose, placebo-controlled erectile dysfunction clinical trial. *BJU International*, 2004. 94(9): 1301-1309.

47. Cetel, N., *Double menopause: what to do when both you and your mate go through hormonal changes together.* 2002, Hoboken, NJ: John Wiley & Sons, Inc.

48. Cheitlin, M.D., Erectile dysfunction: the earliest sign of generalized vascular disease? *J Am Coll Cardiol*, 2004. 43(2): 185-6.

49. Chiurlia, E., et al., Subclinical coronary artery atherosclerosis in patients with erectile dysfunction. *J Am Coll Cardiol*, 2005. 46(8): 1503-6.

50. Comfort, A., *The new joy of sex.* 1991, New York: Crown Publishers, Inc.

51. Corona, G., et al., Aging and pathogenesis of erectile dysfunction. *Int J Impot Res*, 2004. 16(5): 395-402.

52. Costabile, R.A., Optimizing treatment for diabetes mellitus induced erectile dysfunction. *J Urol*, 2003. 170(2 Pt 2): S35-8; discussion S39.

53. Davis, S.R., et al., Endocrine aspects of female sexual dysfunction. *J Sex Med*, 2004. 1(1): 82-6.

54. Dayan, L., et al., A new clinical method for the assessment of penile endothelial function using the flow mediated dilation with plethysmography technique. *J Urol*, 2005. 173(4): 1268-72.

55. de Boer, B.J., et al., The prevalence of bother, acceptance, and need for help in men with erectile dysfunction. *J Sex Med*, 2005. 2(3): 445-50.

56. Dean, J., et al., Psychosocial outcomes and drug attributes affecting treatment choice in men receiving sildenafil citrate and tadalafil for the treatment of erectile dysfunction: results of a multicenter, randomized, open-label, crossover study. *J Sex Med*, 2006. 3: 650-661.

57. DeBusk, R.F., et al., Efficacy and safety of sildenafil citrate in men with erectile dysfunction and stable coronary artery disease. *Am J Cardiol*, 2004. 93(2): 147-53.

58. El-Sakka, A.I., et al., Coronary artery risk factors in patients with erectile dysfunction. *J Urol*, 2004. 172(1): 251-4.

59. Esposito, K., et al., The metabolic syndrome: a cause of sexual dysfunction in women. *Int J Impot Res*, 2005. 17(3): 224-6.

60. Esposito, K., et al., Effect of lifestyle changes on erectile dysfunction in obese men: a randomized controlled trial. *JAMA*, 2004. 291(24): 2978-84.

61. Evans, M.F., Lose weight to lose erectile dysfunction. *Can Fam Physician*, 2005. 51: 47-9.

62. Farnham, A., Is sex necessary? 2003, Forbes.com. http://www.forbes.com/2003/10/08/cz_af_1008health_print.ht ml

63. Fazio, L. and G. Brock, Erectile dysfunction: management update. *CMAJ*, 2004. 170(9): 1429-37.

64. Fedele, D., et al., *Erectile dysfunction in type 1 and type 2 diabetics in Italy.* On behalf of Gruppo Italiano Studio Deficit Erettile nei Diabetici. Int J Epidemiol, 2000. 29(3): 524-31.

65. Fisher, H., *Why we love: the nature and chemistry of romantic love.* 2004, New York: Henry Holt and Company.

66. Fisher, W.A., et al., The multinational Men's Attitudes to Life Events and Sexuality (MALES) Study Phase II: understanding PDE5 inhibitor treatment seeking patterns, among men with erectile dysfunction. *J Sex Med*, 2004. 1(2): 150-60.

67. Fleg, J.L., Physical activity as anti-inflammatory therapy for cardiovascular disease. *Prev Cardiol*, 2005. 8(1): 8-10.

68. Franco, O.H., et al., The Polymeal: a more natural, safer, and probably tastier (than the Polypill) strategy to reduce cardiovascular disease by more than 75%. *BMJ*, 2004. 329(7480): 1447-50.

69. Fung, M.M., R. Bettencourt, and E. Barrett-Connor, Heart disease risk factors predict erectile dysfunction 25 years later: the Rancho Bernardo Study. *J Am Coll Cardiol*, 2004. 43(8): 1405-11.

70. Gazzaruso, C., et al., Relationship between erectile dysfunction and silent myocardial ischemia in apparently uncomplicated type 2 diabetic patients. *Circulation*, 2004. 110(1): 22-6.

71. Ghofrani, H.A., et al., Differences in hemodynamic and oxygenation responses to three different phosphodiesterase-5

inhibitors in patients with pulmonary arterial hypertension: a randomized prospective study. *J Am Coll Cardiol*, 2004. 44(7): 1488-96.

72. Gisquet, V., *Better sex diet.* 2005, Forbes.com. http://www.forbes.com/2005/03/17/cx_vg_0317feat_print.html

73. Goldstein, I., Sexual medicine treatment: lifestyle or life quality? The import of language. *J Sex Med*, 2006. 3(2): 191-3.

74. Goldstein, I., et al., Women's sexual function improves when partners are administered vardenafil for erectile dysfunction: a prospective, randomized, double-blind, placebo-controlled trial. *J Sex Med*, 2005. 2(6): 819-32.

75. Gori, T., et al., Sildenafil prevents endothelial dysfunction induced by ischemia and reperfusion via opening of adenosine triphosphate-sensitive potassium channels: a human in vivo study. *Circulation*, 2005. 111(6): 742-6.

76. Gornik, H.L. and J.A. Beckman, Cardiology patient page. Peripheral arterial disease. *Circulation*, 2005. 111(13): e169-72.

77. Grover, S.A., et al., The prevalence of erectile dysfunction in the primary care setting: importance of risk factors for diabetes and vascular disease. *Arch Intern Med*, 2006. 166(2): 213-9.

78. Hakim, L.S. and D.M. Platt, *The couple's disease: finding a cure for your "lost" love life.* 2002, Delray Beach, FL: DHP Publishers, LLC.

79. Harrar, S. and J. VanTine, Extraordinary togetherness: a woman's guide to love, sex and intimacy. *Prevention Health Books for Women*. 1999, Emmaus, PA: Rodale Inc.

80. Hatzichristou, D., et al., Clinical evaluation and management strategy for sexual dysfunction in men and women. *J Sex Med*, 2004. 1(1): 49-57.

81. Hayes, R. and L. Dennerstein, The impact of aging on sexual function and sexual dysfunction in women: a review of population-based studies. *J Sex Med*, 2005. 2(3): 317-30.

82. Heaton, J.P.W., Hormone treatments and preventive strategies in the aging male: whom and when to treat? *Rev Urol*, 2003. 5 Suppl 1: S16-S21.

83. Heinemann, L.A., et al., Scale for Quality of Sexual Function (QSF) as an outcome measure for both genders? *J Sex Med*, 2005. 2(1): 82-95.

84. Hellstrom, W.J.G., ed. *Male infertility and sexual dysfunction.* 1997, Springer-Verlag: New York.

85. Hellstrom, W.J.G. and M. Kendirci, PDE-5 inhibitors and NAION, in Medscape Urology. 2005. http://www.medscape.com/viewarticle/508658

86. Herrmann, H.C., et al., Can atorvastatin improve the response to sildenafil in men with erectile dysfunction not initially responsive to sildenafil? Hypothesis and pilot trial results. *J Sex Med*, 2006. 3(2): 303-8.

87. Heruti, R., et al., Prevalence of erectile dysfunction among young adults: results of a large-scale survey. *J Sex Med*, 2004. 1(3): 284-91.

88. Hirata, K., et al., Effect of sildenafil on cardiac performance in patients with heart failure. *Am J Cardiol*, 2005. 96(10): 1436-40.

89. Hitti, M., Weight loss may help your sex Life, in *Medscape Today*. 2005. Http://www.medscape.com/viewarticle/ 514784

90. Hooper, A., Anne Hooper's Kama Sutra. 1994, London: Dorling Kindersley.

91. Hooper, A., *K-I-S-S guide to sex.* Keep It Simple Series, ed. J. Williams. 2000, New York: Dorling Kindersley Publishing, Inc.

92. Hutter, A.M., Jr., Role of the cardiologist: clinical aspects of managing erectile dysfunction. *Clin Cardiol*, 2004. 27(4 Suppl 1): 13-7.

93. Hutter, A.M., Jr., Erectile dysfunction and cardiovascular considerations: managing patients effectively with phosphodiesterase type 5 inhibitors. *Clin Cardiol*, 2004. 27(4 Suppl 1): I1-2.

94. Israilov, S., et al., Evaluation of a progressive treatment program for erectile dysfunction in patients with diabetes mellitus. *Int J Impot Res*, 2005. 17(5): 431-6.

95. Jackson, G., Sexual intercourse and stable angina pectoris. *Am J Cardiol*, 2000. 86(2A): 35F-37F.

96. Jackson, G., *Sex, the heart and erectile dysfunction.* 2004, London: Taylor & Francis. 72.

97. Jackson, G., et al., Successful withdrawal of oral long-acting nitrates to facilitate phosphodiesterase type 5 inhibitor use in stable coronary disease patients with erectile dysfunction. *J Sex Med*, 2005. 2(4): 513-6.

98. Kaiser, D.R., et al., Impaired brachial artery endothelium-dependent and independent vasodilation in men with erectile dysfunction and no other clinical cardiovascular disease. *J Am Coll Cardiol*, 2004. 43(2): 179-84.

99. Kemi, O.J., et al., Moderate vs. high exercise intensity: differential effects on aerobic fitness, cardiomyocyte contractility, and endothelial function. *Cardiovasc Res*, 2005. 67(1): 161-72.

100. Kendall, P., Nuts gaining heart-healthy image, in Nutrition News—Colorado State University Cooperative Extension 2002. Http://www.ext.colostate.edu/pubs/ columnnn/nn020225.html

101. Kirby, M., Management of erectile dysfunction in men with cardiovascular conditions. *Br J Cardiol*, 2003. 10(4): 305-307.

102. Kirby, M., *Erectile dysfunction & vascular disease*. 2003, Malden, MA: Blackwell Publishing Ltd. 126.

103. Kloner, R. and H. Padma-Nathan, Erectile dysfunction in patients with coronary artery disease. *Int J Impot Res*, 2005. 17(3): 209-15.

104. Kloner, R.A., Novel phosphodiesterase type 5 inhibitors: assessing hemodynamic effects and safety parameters. *Clin Cardiol*, 2004. 27(4 Suppl 1): 120-5.

105. Kloner, R.A., et al., Erectile dysfunction in the cardiac patient: how common and should we treat? *J Urol*, 2003. 170(2 Pt 2): S46-50; discussion S50.

106. Kostis, J.B., et al., Sexual dysfunction and cardiac risk (the Second Princeton Consensus Conference). *Am J Cardiol*, 2005. 96(12B): 85M-93M.

107. Kratzik, C.W., et al., The impact of age, body mass index and testosterone on erectile dysfunction. *J Urol*, 2005. 174(1): 240-3.

108. Lamm, S. and G.S. Couzens, *The hardness factor. How to achieve your best health and sexual fitness at any age*. 2005, New York: HarperCollins Publishers.

109. Lann, S. and G.S. Couzens, *The hardness factor ™: how to achieve your best health and sexual fitness at any age.* 2005, New York: HarperCollins Publishers.

110. Laumann, E.O., A. Paik, and R.C. Rosen, Sexual dysfunction in the United States: prevalence and predictors. *JAMA*, 1999. 281(6): 537-44.

111. Leiblum, S., et al., Persistent sexual arousal syndrome: a descriptive study. *J Sex Med*, 2005. 2(3): 331-7.

112. Leiblum, S.R. and R.C. Rosen, eds. *Principles and practice of sex therapy: update for the 1990s.* 2nd ed. 1989, The Guilford Press: New York.

113. Lewis, R.W., et al., Epidemiology/risk factors of sexual dysfunction. *J Sex Med*, 2004. 1(1): 35-9.

114. Lue, T.F., et al., Summary of the recommendations on sexual dysfunctions in men. *J Sex Med*, 2004. 1(1): 6-23.

115. Lutz, M.C., et al., Cross-sectional associations of urogenital pain and sexual function in a community based cohort of older men: Olmsted County, Minnesota. *J Urol*, 2005. 174(2): 624-8; discussion 628.

116. Maas, R., et al., The pathophysiology of erectile dysfunction related to endothelial dysfunction and mediators of vascular function. Vasc Med, 2002. 7(3): 213-25.

117. Martin, A.C., It's never too late to start: seven steps toward good health, in *Topics in Advanced Nursing Practice eJournal.* 2002. Http://www.medscape.com/ viewarticle/421471

118. Marwick, T.H., Safe sex for men with coronary artery disease: exercise, sildenafil, and risk of cardiac events. *JAMA*, 2002. 287(6): 766-7.

119. Matsumoto, A.M., Fundamental aspects of hypo-gonadism in the aging male. *Rev Urol*, 2003. 5 Suppl 1: S3-S10.

120. Mazo, E., et al., Testing endothelial function of brachial and cavernous arteries in patients with erectile dysfunction. *J Sex Med*, 2006. 3(2): 323-30.

121. McCullough, A., Case scenarios in androgen deficiency. *Rev Urol*, 2003. 5 Suppl 1: S41-S48.

122. Meston, C. and P. Trapnell, Development and validation of a five-factor sexual satisfaction and distress scale for women: the

Sexual Satisfaction Scale for Women (SSS-W). *J Sex Med*, 2005. 2(1): 66-81.

123. Meston, C.M., Aging and sexuality. *West J Med*, 1997. 167(4): 285-90.

124. Min, J.K., et al., Prediction of coronary heart disease by erectile dysfunction in men referred for nuclear stress testing. *Arch Intern Med*, 2006. 166(2): 201-6.

125. Montague, D.K., et al., Chapter 1: The management of erectile dysfunction: an AUA update. *J Urol*, 2005. 174(1): 230-9.

126. Morales, A., et al., Endocrine aspects of sexual dysfunction in men. *J Sex Med*, 2004. 1(1): 69-81.

127. Moyad, M.A., ed. Preventive medicine and men's health. *Urol Clin North Am*. Vol. 31. 2004.

128. Mulcahy, J.J., ed. *Male sexual function: a guide to clinical management*. 2001, Humana Press: Totowa, NJ.

129. Mulhall, J., et al., Sildenafil citrate response correlates with the nature and the severity of penile vascular insufficiency. *J Sex Med*, 2005. 2(1): 104-8.

130. Munarriz, R., et al., A review of the physiology and pharmacology of peripheral (vaginal and clitoral) female genital arousal in the animal model. *J Urol*, 2003. 170(2 Pt 2): S40-4; discussion S44-5.

131. Nappi, R., et al., Clinical biologic pathophysiologies of women's sexual dysfunction. *J Sex Med*, 2005. 2(1): 4-25.

132. Nehra, A., et al., Third International Conference on the Management of Erectile Dysfunction: Linking Patho- physiology and Therapeutic Response. *J Urol*, 2003. 170(2 Pt 2): S3-5.

133. Nordenberg, T., Looking for a libido lift? The facts about aphrodisiacs. *FDA Consumer*, 1996. 30(1).

134. Oberg, K. and K. Sjogren Fugl-Meyer, On Swedish women's distressing sexual dysfunctions: some concomitant conditions and life satisfaction. *J Sex Med*, 2005. 2(2): 169-80.

135. O'Leary, M.P., Development of an index to evaluate symptoms in men with androgen deficiency. *Rev Urol*, 2003. 5 Suppl 1: S11-S15.

136. Papadopoulos, C., Cardiovascular drugs and sexuality: a cardiologist's review. *Arch Intern Med*, 1980. 140(10): 1341-5.

Bibliography

137. Penedo, F.J. and J.R. Dahn, Exercise and well-being: a review of mental and physical health benefits associated with physical activity. *Curr Opin Psychiatr,* 2005. 18(2): 189-193.

138. Perelman, M., et al., Attitudes of men with erectile dysfunction: a cross-national survey. *J Sex Med,* 2005. 2(3): 397-406.

139. Perricone, N., *The Perricone Weight-Loss Diet: a Simple 3-Part Plan to Lose the Fat, the Wrinkles, and the Years.* 2005, New York: Ballantine Books.

140. Pollifrone, D.L., C.P. Steidle, and S.K. Wilson, *Ending E.D.: a guide to the diagnosis and treatment of erectile dysfunction.* 2001, Fort Wayne, IN: Institute for Urologic Excellence.

141. Polsky, J.Y., et al., Smoking and other lifestyle factors in relation to erectile dysfunction. *BJU Int,* 2005. 96(9): 1355-9.

142. Quirk, F., S. Haughie, and T. Symonds, The use of the sexual function questionnaire as a screening tool for women with sexual dysfunction. *J Sex Med,* 2005. 2(4): 469-77.

143. Rajfer, J., Decreased testosterone in the aging male. *Rev Urol,* 2003. 5 Suppl 1: S1-S2.

144. Rajfer, J., Decreased testosterone in the aging male: summary and conclusions. *Rev Urol,* 2003. 5 Suppl 1: S49-S50.

145. Reeves, M.J. and A.P. Rafferty, Healthy lifestyle characteristics among adults in the United States, 2000. *Arch Intern Med,* 2005. 165(8): 854-7.

146. Reinberg, S., Oysters may be an aphrodisiac after all. 2005, MSN.com. Http://health.msn.com/centers/men sexualhealth/articlepage.aspx?cp-documentid=100101156

147. Rosen, R., et al., Sensitivity of the psychological and interpersonal relationship scales to oral therapies for erectile dysfunction. *J Sex Med,* 2005. 2(4): 461-8.

148. Rosen, R.C., et al., The multinational Men's Attitudes to Life Events and Sexuality (MALES) study: I. Prevalence of erectile dysfunction and related health concerns in the general population. *Curr Med Res Opin,* 2004. 20(5): 607-17.

149. Rosenfeld, I., Heart health starts with you. *Parade,* 2005.

150. Rosenfeld, I., *Dr. Isadore Rosenfeld's 2005 breakthrough health. Up-to-the minute medical news you need to know.* 2005, Emmaus, PA: Rodale Inc. 281.

151. Rosenthal, S.H., *Sex over 40.* 1999, New York: Tarcher/Putnam.

152. Saenz de Tejada, I., et al., Physiology of erectile function. *J Sex Med*, 2004. 1(3): 254-65.

153. Saigal, C.S., et al., Predictors and prevalence of erectile dysfunction in a racially diverse population. *Arch Intern Med*, 2006. 166(2): 207-12.

154. Salonia, A., et al., Chocolate and women's sexual health: an intriguing correlation. *J Sex Med*, 2006. 3: 476-482.

155. Saltzman, E.A., A.T. Guay, and J. Jacobson, Improvement in erectile function in men with organic erectile dysfunction by correction of elevated cholesterol levels: a clinical observation. *J Urol*, 2004. 172(1): 255-8.

156. Sasayama, S., et al., Men's Health Study: epidemiology of erectile dysfunction and cardiovascular disease. *Circ J*, 2003. 67(8): 656-9.

157. Seftel, A.D., Phosphodiesterase type 5 inhibitor different- iation based on selectivity, pharmacokinetic, and efficacy profiles. *Clin Cardiol*, 2004. 27(4 Suppl 1): I14-19.

158. Seftel, A.D., et al., eds. *Sexual dysfunction: male and female*. 2004, Mosby: New York. 312.

159. Sehgal, V.N. and G. Srivastava, *Erectile dysfunctions. Skinmed*, 2003. 2(6): 350-6.

160. Shabsigh, R., *Back to great sex: overcome ED and reclaim lost intimacy*. 2002, New York: Kensington Publishing Corp.

161. Sharlip, I.D., PDE5 inhibitors do not cause NAION. *J Sex Med*, 2006. 3 Suppl 2: 80.

162. Sheehy, G., *Sex and the seasoned woman: pursuing the passionate life*. 2006, New York: Random House.

163. Shindel, A., et al., Sexual dysfunction in female partners of men who have undergone radical prostatectomy correlates with sexual dysfunction of the male partner. *J Sex Med*, 2005. 2(6): 833-41; discussion 841.

164. Shiri, R., et al., Relationship between smoking and erectile dysfunction. *Int J Impot Res*, 2005. 17(2): 164-9.

165. Shiri, R., et al., Effect of lower urinary tract symptoms on the incidence of erectile dysfunction. *J Urol*, 2005. 174(1): 205-9; discussion 209.

166. Shiri, R., et al., Effect of life-style factors on incidence of erectile dysfunction. *Int J Impot Res*, 2004. 16(5): 389-94.

167. Siebert, D., Sexual health: counseling in primary care, in *Medscape Today* - National Conference for Nurse Practitioners 2001. 2001. Http://www.medscape.com/viewprogram/852_childindex

168. Siroky, M.B. and K.M. Azadzoi, Vasculogenic erectile dysfunction: newer therapeutic strategies. *J Urol*, 2003. 170(2 Pt 2): S24-9; discussion S29-30.

169. Smith, K.M. and F. Romanelli, Recreational use and misuse of phosphodiesterase 5 inhibitors. *J Am Pharm Assoc* (Wash DC), 2005. 45(1): 63-72; quiz 73-5.

170. Solomon, H., J.W. Man, and G. Jackson, Erectile dysfunction and the cardiovascular patient: endothelial dysfunction is the common denominator. *Heart*, 2003. 89(3): 251-3.

171. Somers, S., *The sexy years: discover the hormone connection: the secret to fabulous sex, great health, and vitality, for men and women.* 2004, New York: Crown Publishers.

172. SoRelle, R., At the heart of the matter: sex. *Circulation*, 1999. 100(21): e102-3.

173. Steers, W.D., Viability and safety of combination drug therapies for erectile dysfunction. *J Urol*, 2003. 170(2 Pt 2): S20-3; discussion S23.

174. Steidle, C.P., *The impotence sourcebook.* 1999, Chicago: Lowell House/NTC/Contemporary Publishing Group, Inc.

175. Steidle, C.P., *Testosterone: a user's manual.* 2001, Fort Wayne, IN: Christopher P. Steidle, publisher. 130.

176. Steidle, C.P., New advances in the treatment of hypogonadism in the aging male. *Rev Urol*, 2003. 5 Suppl 1: S34-S40.

177. Stern, S., Symptoms other than chest pain may be important in the diagnosis of "silent ischemia," or "the sounds of silence". *Circulation*, 2005. 111(24): e435-7.

178. Sun, P. and R. Swindle, Are men with erectile dysfunction more likely to have hypertension than men without erectile dysfunction? A naturalistic national cohort study. *J Urol*, 2005. 174(1): 244-8.

179. Sztajzel, J., et al., Effect of sexual activity on cycle ergometer stress test parameters, on plasmatic testosterone levels and on concentration capacity. A study in high-level male athletes

performed in the laboratory. *J Sports Med Phys Fitness*, 2000. 40(3): 233-9.

180. Tariq, S.H. and J.E. Morley, Maintaining sexual function in older women: physical impediments and psychosocial issues. *Women's Health in Primary Care*, 2003. 6(3): 157-162.

181. Tenover, J.L., The androgen-deficient aging male: current treatment options. *Rev Urol*, 2003. 5 Suppl 1: S22-S28.

182. Thethi, T.K., N.O. Asafu-Adjaye, and V.A. Fonseca, Erectile dysfunction. *Clin Diabetes*, 2005. 23(3): 105-113.

183. Thompson, I.M., et al., Erectile dysfunction and subsequent cardiovascular disease. *JAMA*, 2005. 294(23): 2996-3002.

184. Tikiz, C., et al., Sexual dysfunction in female subjects with fibromyalgia. *J Urol*, 2005. 174(2): 620-3.

185. Valli, G. and E.G. Giardina, Benefits, adverse effects and drug interactions of herbal therapies with cardiovascular effects. *J Am Coll Cardiol*, 2002. 39(7): 1083-95.

186. Van Gaal, L.F., et al., Effects of the cannabinoid-1 receptor blocker rimonabant on weight reduction and cardiovascular risk factors in overweight patients: 1-year experience from the RIO-Europe study. *Lancet*, 2005. 365(9468): 1389-97.

187. Vega, C., Weight loss helpful in obese men with erectile dysfunction, in Medscape Today—CME. 2004. Http://www.medscape.com/viewarticle/481470

188. Wagner, G., et al., Ethical aspects of sexual medicine. *J Sex Med*, 2005. 2(2): 163-8.

189. Webster, L.J., et al., Use of sildenafil for safe improvement of erectile function and quality of life in men with New York Heart Association classes II and III congestive heart failure: a prospective, placebo-controlled, double-blind crossover trial. *Arch Intern Med*, 2004. 164(5): 514-20.

190. Weijmar Schultz, W., et al., Women's sexual pain and its management. *J Sex Med*, 2005. 2(3): 301-16.

191. Yaman, O., et al., The effect of diabetes mellitus treatment and good glycemic control on the erectile function in men with diabetes mellitus-induced erectile dysfunction: a pilot study. *J Sex Med*, 2006. 3(2): 344-8.

192. Yassin, A.A., Brain sex—testosterone role in personality evolution; females and males are different? *J Sex Med*, 2006. 3 Suppl 2: 81-82.

193. Yu, S. and J.W.G. Yarnell, Exercise for the prevention of cardiovascular disease: how vigorous and how often? *Cardiovasc Rev Rep*, 2004. 25(6): 274-276.

194. Zhang, X.H., et al., Testosterone restores diabetes-induced erectile dysfunction and sildenafil responsive- ness in two distinct animal models of chemical diabetes. *J Sex Med*, 2006. 3(2): 253-64; discussion 264-5, author reply 265-6.

Index

Glucophage XR, 31
glucose, 27
  see also blood glucose, 27
  laboratory tests, 67
glucose meters, 31
glycemic control, 30, 31, 49, 80
gonadal dysfunction, 28
good fats, 118, 119
growth hormone, 120
Guide for Quitting Smoking, 121
gynocomastia, 54

H
habanera peppers, 127
hair growth, 47, 141
hardening of the arteries, 7
  see also atherosclerosis
Hardness Factor, The, 128
HCTZ, 42
HDL good cholesterol, 32–35,
  37, 126
  see also high-density lipopro-
    tein level (HDL
head of penis
  see glans, 20
head trauma, 20
headaches, 39, 76
health history, 62
healthful diet, 36, 115-120
healthful fats, 33
heart
  electrical activity testing, 72
heart anatomy, 105
heart attacks, 18, 39, 55
heart beat
  irregular, or increased, 17
heart disease, 6, 13, 17, 18, 28,
  114, 119
heart failure I, 103
heart-healthy eating plan, 44
heart rate, 106
  decreasers, 42
heart surgery
  and sexual activity, 106
heart valve, 107
heart valve disease
  and sexual activity, 107
hematoma, 95
hemoglobin A1c, 29

test, 29
hemorrhoids, 135
hepatitis, 56
herbal remedies, 65
heredity
  as a factor in cholesterol
    levels, 33
hernias, 93
high blood pressure, 15, 18,
  20, 30, 56, 64, 103
  early warning signs, 44
  see also hypertension
  and sexual activity, 104
  medications, 41–44
  symptomless, 39
high blood sugar, 15
  levels, 28
high cholesterol, 10, 30
high cholesterol levels, 32
high-density lipoprotein level
  (HDL), 15, 32, 34, 35
  levels, 35
high lipids, 32
  see also cholesterol
high-risk cardiac patients,
  102–104
high total cholesterol, 32
height loss, 53
hormonal imbalances, 28
hormone deficiency, 135
hormones, 15, 17, 21, 32, 40,
  68
  growth, 120
  testing, 138
hot flashes, 140
House Resolution 1903, 98
Hydodiuril, 42
hydrochlorthiazide, 42
hydrogenated oils, 118
Hygroton, 42
hypercholsterolemia, 32
  see also high cholesterol
    levels
hypertension, 13, 17, 18, 28,
  30, 39–45, 67
  ability to achieve orgasm,
    18
  arousal, 18
  as a cause of ED, 40, 110

About the Authors

Christopher P. Steidle, M.D., is a board-certified urologist in private practice at Northeast Indiana Urology, Fort Wayne, Indiana. He's also a clinical associate professor of urology at the Indiana University School of Medicine. Dr. Steidle has been actively involved in clinical research since 1989, specializing in male and female sexual dysfunction as well as urinary incontinence, prostate cancer, and infectious diseases. He is the founder and principal investigator of Northeast Indiana Research, LLC, a nationally recognized research facility.

Dr. Steidle graduated magna cum laude from Tulane University, New Orleans, with a bachelor of science degree in parasitology. He received his medical degree from the University of Virginia School of Medicine.

A consultant and lecturer on sexual dysfunction and prostate disease, Dr. Steidle has authored more than forty-six peer-reviewed publications and is the author of *Sex and the Heart*, (First Edition, 2006), *The Impotence Source Book* (1999) and *Testosterone: A User's Manual* (2001).

J anet Casperson, BS, MSN, ANP-C, is a board-certified nurse practitioner at Northeast Indiana Urology, where she is Sexual Health Director. For more than twenty years she has treated patients for cardiovascular disease and sexual dysfunction.

Ms. Casperson graduated from Perdue University with a bachelor of science degree in nursing degree and a master's degree in nursing from Ball State University. She is a member of Sigma Theta Tau International Honor Society of Nursing. She's also a member of the Sexual Medicine Society, and has been a presenter at annual meetings, a s well as at national nurse practitioner meetings.

She has served on the clinical faculty at St. Francis University, Ball State University, and Perdue University. She has been a guest lecturer on Sex and the Heart at the International Congress of Cognitive Psychotherapy, Rome, Italy.

Ms. Casperson has served as a consultant to patient support groups and to sexual health clinics across the United States; she has also been a medical advisor to national magazines. She is co-author of *Sex and the Heart* (First Edition, 2006).

Consumer Health Titles from Addicus Books
Visit our online catalog at www.addicusbooks.com

Simple Changes—
   The Boomer's Guide to a Healthier, Happier Life. . . . $9.95
A Simple Guide to Thyroid Disorders. $14.95
Straight Talk About Breast Cancer—
   From Diagnosis to Recovery $15.95
The Stroke Recovery Book—
   A Guide for Patients and Families $14.95
The Surgery Handbook—
   A Guide to Understanding Your Operation $14.95
Understanding Lumpectomy—
   A Treatment Guide for Breast Cancer. $14.95
Understanding Parkinson's Disease—A Self-Help Guide . . $14.95
Understanding Peyronie's Disease $16.95
Understanding Your Living Will $12.95
Your Complete Guide to Breast Augmentation
   & Body Contouring $21.95
Your Complete Guide to Breast Reduction & Breast Lifts . $21.95
Your Complete Guide to Facial Cosmetic Surgery $19.95
Your Complete Guide to Facelifts $21.95
Your Complete Guide to Nose Reshaping. $21.95

Book Order Form

Please send:

_____copies of _____

at_____each.

Total   _____

Nebraska residents add 6.5% sales tax   _____

Shipping/Handling   _____

$5.00 postage for first book: _____

$1.20 for each additional book: _____

TOTAL ENCLOSED_____

Name _____

Address_____

City _____State _____Zip _____

□ Visa   □ Mastercard   □ American Express   □ Discover

Credit card number_____

Expiration date _____

Ways to Order:

- Mailorder by credit card, personal check, or money order.
  Send to: Addicus Books, P.O. Box 45327, Omaha, NE 68145

- **Order TOLL FREE:** 800-352-2873

- **Visit us online at:** www.AddicusBooks.com

- **For discounts on bulk purchases, call our Special Sales Dept. at (402) 330-7493**